THREE TURNS OF A KALEIDOSCOPE

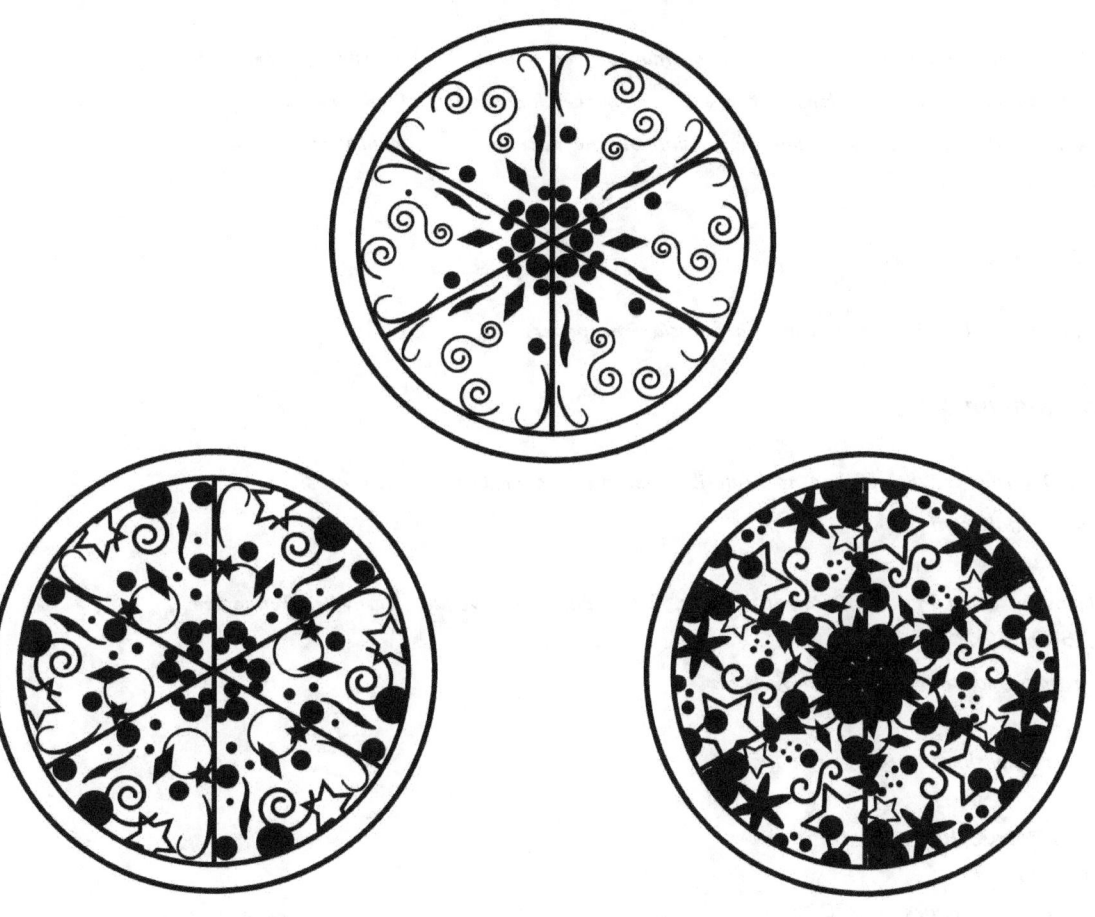

HEALING THE VICTIM WITHIN

BONNIE SUZANNE JOHNSON

WESTVIEW PUBLISHING CO., INC., NASHVILLE, TENNESSEE

© 2008 by Bonnie Suzanne Johnson.

All Rights Reserved. No portion of this book may be reproduced in any fashion, either mechanically or electronically, without the express written permission of the author. Short excerpts may be used with the permission of the author or the publisher for the purposes of media reviews.

Second Edition, October 2019

Printed in the United States of America on acid-free paper.

ISBN 978-0-9819172-3-8

Bonnie S. Johnson can be reached at healerjbonnie@me.com or through her website: www.healerjbonnie.com

Illustrations by Brian Parker of Parker Designs, 2416 Eastland Avenue, Nashville, Tennessee 37206, 615-262-7400.
   prkrdsgns@aol.com or parkerdesigns.biz

Prepress by Published by Westview, Inc.

IDEAS INTO BOOKS: WESTVIEW®
P.O. Box 605
Kingston Springs, Tennessee 37082
www.publishedbywestview.com

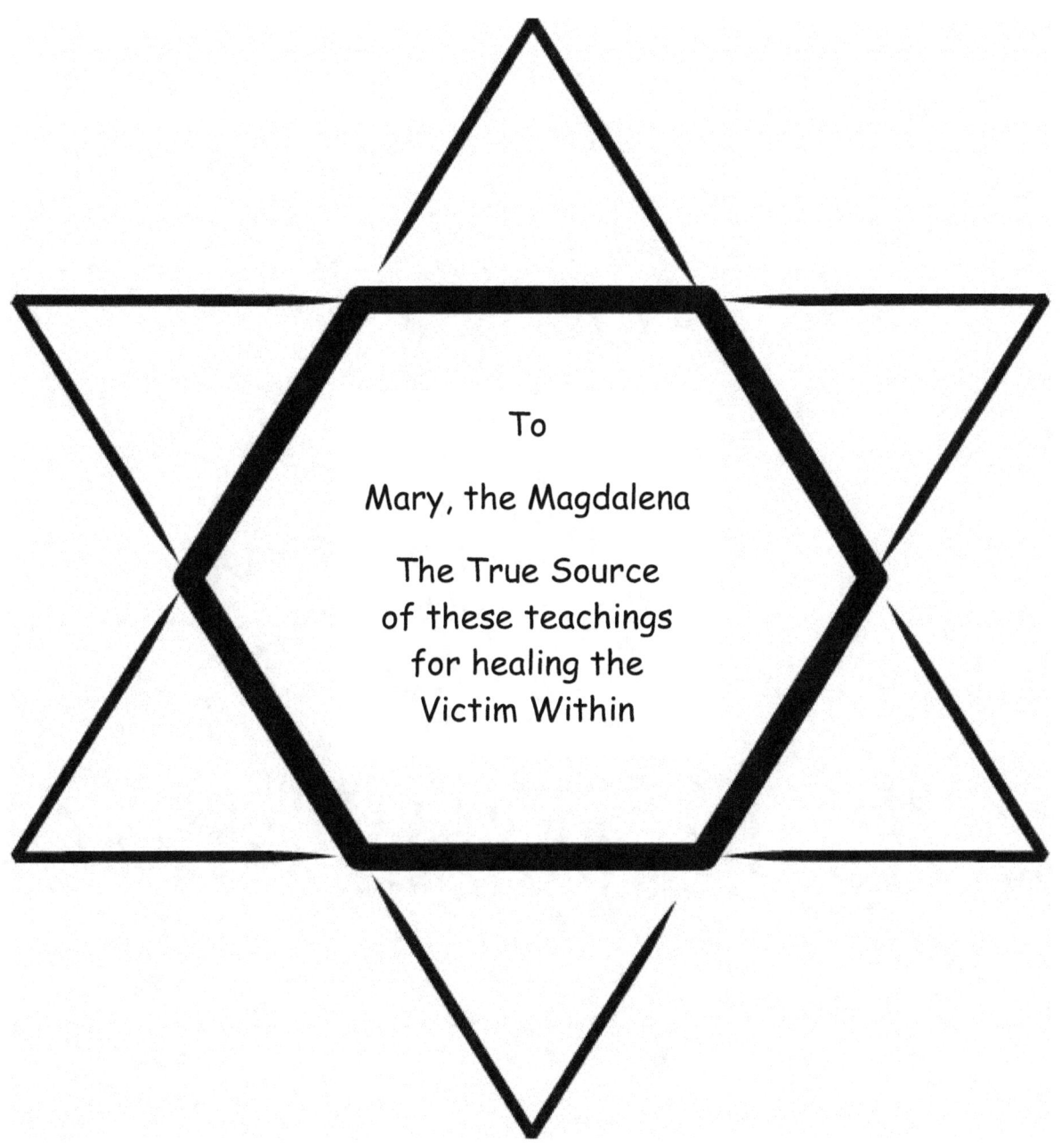

CONTENTS

GRATITUDE 1

INTRODUCTION 3
    The Cries of the Inner Victim 4
    Victim in the Making 5
    Seeking a Change 6
    Receiving Guidance That Heals 7
    Preponderance of Triangles 9
    Get It to Them 10
    Guidelines For Using This Book 11
    Definitions 13
    Pointers 15

Part I: HARNESSING COSMIC ENERGIES 17

Memoirs 18

Why Triangles? 19
    The Characteristics and Qualities of Triangles 20
    The Power of Three's 22
    The Cosmic Influence of the Six-Pointed Star 24
    Summary 26

Brief Overview 27

Prep One: Accessing Healing Energies 29
    The Six-Pointed Star: A Healing Meditation 30
    Star's Six Spiritual Qualities
        through the Eyes of the Human Energy System 32
    Review and Summary of Prep One 33

Part II: INNOCENCE 35

Prep Two: Recalling the Natural Mammal 37
    Memoirs...37
    Meet Your Healthy Natural Mammal 38
    Snapshots of the Natural Mammal....................................40
    Survival: a Celebration..43
    Natural Mammal through the Eyes of the Human Energy System......44
    Review and Summary of Prep Two 46

Part III: SEPARATION.. 47

Memoirs..48

From Natural Mammal to Drama Dance 51

Prep Three: Choosing a Drama Dance Experience 55
    Sample Prep Three 56
    Tips for Identifying the Three Roles..................................59
    The Drama Dance: What is it? 60
    Process of Becoming a Member of Three-Stepping Drama Dance Club....62
    The Attraction and Perpetuation of the Drama Dance..........68
    Complete or Modify Prep Three.......................................70
    Review and Summary of Prep Three 70

Part IV: INITIATION 71

Memoirs 72

Three Turns: Three Healing Triangles 75

Stop Paying Your Dues: The Way Out
    Resigning Membership in the Drama Dance Club 76

First Turn: Becoming Safe 79
    Need-Help-Action Triangle
        through the Eyes of the Human Energy System 80
    How to Use Need-Help-Action Triangle for Healing 82
    Pointers 83
    Review and Summary of First Turn 85

Second Turn: Shifting Awareness to Learning 89
    Student-Teacher-Knowledge Triangle
        through Eyes of Human Energy System 90
    Pointers 91
    How to use Student-Teacher-Knowledge Triangle for Healing 92
    Review and Summary of the Second Turn 94

Third Turn: Transforming to Living Anew 97
    Death-Birth-Life Triangle
        through the Eyes of the Human Energy System 98
    How to Use Death-Birth-Life Triangle for Healing 99
    Review and Summary of Third Turn 102

Six Spiritual Qualities 103
    Truth 105
    Self-Love with Memoirs 106
    Forgiveness with Memoirs 108
    Wisdom 110
    Compassion with Memoirs 111
    Higher Purpose 113
    Summary 114

Part V: RETURN TO WHOLENESS 115

Part VI: RESOURCES 117

Energetic Support System 119
- Amygdala Connection 121
- Brain Connection 124
- Chakra Correspondence 125
- Quieting Hyper-Arousal of Fight-or-Flight 126
- Shift-of-Consciousness Breathing 127
- Tapping for Changing Habitual Hyper-arousal Reactions 128
- Three Gates and Three Cauldrons 129
- Rosa Mystica Meditation 132

Personal Stories of Healing the Victim Within 133
1. An Old Story: Yamina 135
2. Dramatic Food: Rene 142
3. A Love Story: Melodie 153

Quick! What's Your First Thought? 161

Complete Step-By-Step Overview 165

Bibliography 173

ACKNOWLEDGEMENTS 177

ABOUT THE AUTHOR 179

GRATITUDE

I am deeply indebted to Karla Kincannon and Nelson Villalobos for the many hours of discussions, clarifications, and tweakings in the early days as the ideas contained in this book were developing. I remember well how we cut paper triangles, turning them this way and that! Their thought-gifts are threads woven throughout these writings.

To Lois Schmidt and Martha Rather, who willingly bared their souls as we applied the Healing-The-Victim-Within teachings (over and over!), and who gave tantalizing and challenging feedback, Namaste[1].

My deepest gratitude to the students of the Healing Touch Review classes in Nashville, Tennessee, who enthusiastically explored these ideas and healing approaches in their embryonic stages, during intense labor, birth, and exhilarating infancy. Patricia Barlow, Tom Barron, Mary Ann Bennett, Carol Bevis, Kim Crowe, Linda Doochin, Michael Doochin, Linda Hunt, Ronna Seibert, Deanna Smith, Betty Stadler, Barbara Tomlinson: you all are the best midwives any birther could ask for!

To all the clients, whose life journeys I have been blessed to be part of and to remember together that we are indeed whole and holy, thank you for opening your hearts and souls in my presence.

To my mother, the extraordinary priestess disguised as an ordinary housewife, thank you for keeping watch over the ancient cauldron. Through you I learned of the "old ways" shrouded beneath a kitchen apron.

To Mary, the Magdalena, eternal reverence for allowing me to be the cauldron in which these teachings fermented and distilled.

---

[1] Namaste is said to another person as a way to recognize the divine in that person and thus, communicate a deep respect. The word is derived from the ancient Sanskrit language of India.

INTRODUCTION

Every particle of the world is a mirror. In each
atom blazes forth the light of a thousand suns.
                                    Mahmud Shabistari [2]

Into my outstretched hand, my older friend places a long and colorful cylinder. With an expectant smile, she directs: "Look through the hole on the end." Puzzled and curious, I peer through the pea-sized opening. Dark shadows greet me. "Raise the other end toward the light and turn the dial," instructs my friend. As the light from the lamp seeps through and I turn the dial, the dark shadows shift and become a bright mandala. Intrigued, I point the tube toward a brighter light and rotate the dial. Tiny pieces of colored material rearrange themselves to reveal a new image. The delight of the emerging beauty sends me looking for more as I point it toward the morning sun. With another twist of the dial, a new design stuns me into quiet pleasure.

My childhood encounter with a kaleidoscope—from dark shadows to light infused images to quiet pleasure—mirrors this book's process for healing the internalized Victim. When we find ourselves immersed in the shadowy replays of past experiences that adversely affect our present life, this healing process encourages us to point our metaphorical kaleidoscope toward the light. As we turn the dial, the bits of information reorder themselves and reveal a new image and a new perspective. Seeking more awareness, we search for greater light. Enhanced illumination and another turn provides a shift in perspective that frees us from repetitive and hurt-filled thoughts and behaviors. Surprised, we soon notice ourselves enjoying soothing contentment.

Without light or movement, a particular pattern remains static and hidden. The bits and pieces of these troubling past experiences create a disturbing and enduring pattern of relating to oneself and to others as an inner Victim. Over and over, we view these long ago experiences the same way. Living through a narrow perspective of gloomy silhouettes—without the benefit of light or movement—we remain stuck in the past.

---

[2] From "The Mirror" in the *Secret Rose Garden* by the medieval Sufi poet Mahmud Shabistari

Strangely, our past experiences reconstructed as inner Victims can be the proverbial tap on the shoulder that starts us searching for fuller and brighter perspectives and new images of our past and of our present selves.

The Cries of the Inner Victim

The Victim within us can be heard in our own voices when we grumble: "Poor me! Nothing ever goes right for me." We beseech: "Why am I to blame for everything that goes wrong?" We whine: "Why do people treat me so badly? Why don't people appreciate the good things I do for them?" We desperately want to know: "Why am I so miserable? Why is my life one big drama after another?"

When we ask these questions, this is our inner Victim crying out for help. Too often we find ourselves caught in the frenzy of High Drama and we don't know how we got there or how to change what is happening.

The experience of the Victim within is not a new phenomenon. We even find the Victim in our sacred stories. In the tradition of the people of Abraham and Sarai, the first man and first woman were innocent, easy going, provided for and protected in the Garden of Eden. Everything changed when they ate the forbidden fruit. When confronted about their illicit behavior, both personify the Victim when they deny responsibility for their actions, shifting the blame to others for their shame-filled plight.

Just as in the Garden of Eden, once upon a time the whole of us was playful, capable, powerful, innocent, and vulnerable. Along life's journey, we too became separated from our idyllic beginnings. We began to live through the perceptions of our inner Victim, the aspects of us who believe and behave as if we are helpless and powerless. For a variety of reasons—from trauma to socialization—we humans sometimes assume the role of Victim, even when we have the power to change our current situation.

Victim in the Making

The distress, which contributed to the Victim within me, began early in my life. One disturbing event transpired when I was nine years old. My older sister Pam and I had just finished performing at a formal piano recital. Jumping up and down with excitement, I cried out: "Mom! Mom! Look, I got excellent!" I held my head high and my hands stretched upward as I danced a little victory jig. I knew I had played my piece with precision and perfection—no mistakes. Confirming this was a large-sized EXCELLENT written across the certificate I waved in front of my mother's face. She barely looked at it or me. Instead, she chastised: "Bonnie, you may have gotten EXCELLENT because you played all the notes correctly and Pam only got VERY GOOD because she made a few mistakes but her playing was full of emotion. She put her heart into it. You didn't. Pam deserved an excellent more than you." My powerful and excited self was crushed and confused.

I lost my excitement about piano playing and I carried the hurt of her words into my adult years. I frequently replayed the scene in my mind, re-experiencing afresh the pain of her words and the loss of my excited powerful and able self. Each time I replayed the scene, I was seeking a new ending, seeking a different way in which my mother responded to my excellent piano playing. My thoughts often went to: Why couldn't she have hugged me and told me she was proud of me? Why didn't she say I did a great job? These thoughts were my attempt to change the past and restore my excited self.

I continue to try to restore my excited self in the following scenario. When I was twenty-two, my parents and younger siblings went to Canada for a vacation. I was left home alone in the emptiness created by their leaving. Restless, I looked for something to do. Soon the shelves in the over-sized pantry were emptied and I was deep into sorting and rearranging my mother's domain. Over several days everything was scrubbed clean and put back in its rightful—according to me—place. As I worked, I imagined my mother coming into the house, surprised and pleased at the conversion from mess to tidiness. I patted myself on the back for coming up with such a brilliant idea for doing something nice for my mother. When my family returned I barely let them in the house before I pulled my mother down the hall and through the dining room to the pantry. My face was full of smiles and my body trembled with the anticipation of her pleasure. As soon as my mother saw her transformed pantry, she scowled and blasted me with incendiary words. She was furious with me for changing her workspace.

My mother did not perceive my good intentions and I did not understand what I had done wrong. In one second, all my expectations turned inside out. Where I anticipated her praise and gratitude, I now received her scorn and displeasure. I was deeply hurt; I saw my mother as mean and ungrateful. I swore I would never again clean anything in her house. I had no idea what went wrong and felt helpless and hopeless to reclaim my happiness. I was stuck in my misery.

These are just two of the countless experiences in which I lose my powerful and joy-filled self and become dejected and trapped with no awareness on how to change. In the midst of these losses, I felt helpless and acted as if I was a Victim of events beyond my control. There is a Rwandan saying which advises: "You can outdistance that which is running after you, but not what is running inside you." I spent years trying to get as much distance from the misery, confusion and shame running inside me. Often I asked: "Why is life always in an uproar? Why does life have to be this way?" Caught in the web of obsessive hashing and re-hashing self-criticism, I didn't know how I got there or how to change what was happening. However, I did realize I was miserable and I wanted my life to be better.

Seeking a Change

In my search for a way out of this misery, information about the inner Victim crisscrossed my life in multiple ways. Books, conversations and personal struggles kept bringing it into my awareness. The Karpman Drama Triangle[3], one of the best descriptions of this internalization of the Victim and the ensuing misery-producing interactions, first came to my attention in my own personal counseling sessions back in the 1970's. I was re-introduced in an academic setting through graduate classes in counseling and child development, and later in continuing education study of hands-on energetic healing and holistic nursing.

---
3 First described and labeled by Stephen Karpman, MD in 1970's, this is a model for depicting complex human interactions that include high drama and misery.

In designing the Drama Triangle, Dr. Stephen Karpman, a teacher of Transactional Analysis[4], used a simple diagram of a triangle to depict a complex model of human interactions. Karpman's descriptions of the three roles—Victim, Rescuer and Persecutor[5]—as they are acted out in the Drama, helped me to notice how frequently I, my family, friends, clients and people I encountered casually in stores, on planes, and at meetings, related to each other as self-appointed, self-perceived Victims, bumbling Rescuers, and emotionally devastating Persecutors.

Through an ongoing scrutiny of the inner Victim, I became aware that much is written and taught that describes the Drama Triangle and its quick changing roles. However, little was available that gave specific ways to <u>heal</u> a high Drama way of relating. As a nurse healer, I started exploring ways to heal this futile and addictive cycle.

Receiving Guidance That Heals

I learned how to meditate from my mother who would have rivaled any Zen master in her methodology. When I was toddler and barely able to sit comfortably, I was given the assignment to sit on the "pot" until I had produced something. I knew better than to get up before I had. The lightning quick strike of a Zen master was no match for one of my mother's "looks." So I whiled away the time by way of musings. Soon I was deep in contemplation. Creative inspirations would come to me in that meditative state.

Our downstairs bathroom was cramped; the toilet faced the sink with little room between. At three years old, I sat with my legs swinging free off the floor and bumping easily into the sink. Quiet reigned there, away from the bustle of a house full of brothers and sisters, parents and grandparents, cats and dogs. There, without interruptions, I talked with Mary, an invisible Being. I listened,

---

[4] A system of psychotherapy with a starting premise of "I'm OK. You're OK." Transactional Analysis is the brain child of psychologist Eric Berne of Games People Play

[5] Victim, with a capital V, is one that is acted on and adversely affected by an internal force or agent, usually one's feelings, thoughts and beliefs.. Rescuer is one who helps or takes care of another or oneself when such help or care is not needed and sometimes is actually harmful. A Persecutor is one who harasses in a manner designed to injure, grieve or afflict self or another who has the means to defend and does not.

rapt and wrapped in a mystical communication. My face tilted upward and cocked slightly to the left, my eyes widened, and my ears sparked. As a strong vibration entered me, my mouth formed the round O of surprise and enchantment. Her surrounding Light imbued me with Knowing.

My early experiences of meditation and the accompanying conversations with Mary began a lifetime of communications with Divine Presence that has guided me in my daily life. The name for this Presence has changed throughout the years but the quieting and awareness has remained constant. Whether I call this quieting, stillness, meditation, contemplative or centering prayer, I experience a deep and profound connection with a loving and enlightening Presence. When I started studying hands-on energetic healing in the 1980's, this continuing guidance informed and supported me as I provided healings for others.

I live in a brick and stucco house that sits atop a wind brushed hill in a peaceful, tree rich neighborhood. On the same property is a small building that serves as my holistic nursing and healing office. The surrounding tall pine and cedar, shrubby St John's Wort, and delicate dogwoods seem to pour their verdant abundance through the office windows and into the healing rooms. The lush green contrasts and enlivens the faint lilac of the inside walls. Here, in 1997, I sat immersed in the vibrancy of nature's energetic support and went into a deep meditative state. I became aware of the Divine Presence of invisible helpers—angelic, shamanic, spiritual and familiar—who guide and support me. The most familiar, for She and I have been conversing since I was a toddler, is the invisible being whom I now know as Mary, the Magdalena. As the vibration I recognized as Mary began to flow into and through me, I asked Mary how do we do this; how do we heal this dramatic and troubling pattern of humans relating as if we are powerless and helpless Victims? How do we heal this virtual Drama Dance[6]? How do we heal the internal turmoil, which spurs us to run?

The answers—received in numerous meditations and over a period of several years—became a multi-faceted process for healing the internalized Victim. Called *Three Turns of a Kaleidoscope*, it is an intentional coming together of sacred geometry[7], energetic healing techniques, and incisive questions. The spiritual energies, received through this healing process, transform and

---

[6] An internalization as oneself as Victim and subsequent misery-producing drama-like interactions.

[7] Sacred Geometry is the intentional use of numbers and shapes to bring in higher vibrational energies for healing and heightened awareness.

transcend the Drama and are meant for all of us who find ourselves embroiled in the frenzy and misery of dramatic dancing **and** are ready to give up the Drama, ready to restore our living as the whole and holy beings we are.

Preponderance of Triangles

Often the guided information from Mary would come in bits and pieces. At other times it would gush out as if a dam had burst. Then I would receive no more information for months. Suddenly another dam would break and out would pour a seemingly unending stream. Sometimes a nugget would appear and instantly other information would all click together. At times I did nothing; it just seemed to sit inside me, simmering, for months on end.

In 2003, I received Mary's guided directions for using the geometric and energetic form of the six-pointed star as a healing meditation. A few weeks later, I was looking through papers and files when I happened upon paper triangles with words written in each of the corners. These paper triangles were my notes of guided information—received five years before—put in a folder—to gather dust while the information mixed and fermented within me. As I perused these cryptic messages, scales fell off my eyes and I saw how it all fit together.

A total of seven triangles are used in this healing process. Two triangles, one facing down and one up, interlace to make the six-pointed star for the healing meditation. The common space—a hexagram—shared by both triangles, creates an energetic portal through which powerful healing energies become available for healing the Victim within. A third triangle accesses our natural mammal energies (that is who we were before we learned this skewed way of Dancing). The fourth triangle is the one that Karpman used to depict the drama interactions. The fifth, sixth and seventh triangles are the three turns of a kaleidoscope and contain the information laid out on the dusty paper triangles.

Inside a kaleidoscope, three long mirrors are positioned in a triangular shape to create triple reflections. The triple mirrors reflect tiny pieces of colored material to form patterns that change as the kaleidoscope turns. When the mirrors are clear and intact, the orderly designs are beautiful; when cracked or cloudy, the designs are muddled. The Drama is one such muddled design, whose tiny particles reflect off fractured mirrors to create a distressing pattern. When kept dark and stagnant, the drama pattern persists. When an intact kaleidoscope is pointed toward the light, the first, then the second, and finally the third turn rearranges those same tiny particles to reveal new and heightened perceptions. As we will learn in the following pages, these new perceptions, acquired through the three turns of the kaleidoscope, reflect back the transformation and subsequent healing of the Victim within us.

Get It to Them

When I was ready to use the information, I tested the teachings by first applying them to my own life. Then I shared them with my healer friends. As I became more acquainted with the teachings and specific healing techniques, I brought my mushrooming knowledge to the healing students I supervised in weekly classes. Soon, my clients began to hear about what I was doing and they asked for the information and to receive the hands-on-healing techniques.

The fermentation of all these teachings began to bubble over. Not sure what I was to do with this overflowing pot, I took some time apart to meditate, read and just be with the material. One day, after a few days of reading and writing and studying, I sat outdoors overlooking the bluff in Sewanee, Tennessee, and went into deep meditation. In the powerful voice of Mary, the Magdalena, I was admonished: "Put down those books, quit studying this over and over and go teach it. People are in need of this—get it to them."

The first workshop, titled "Healing The Inner Victim," was taught to a focus group made up of fifteen seasoned healers. Subsequent workshops have continued to substantiate the direction: "People are in need of this—get it to them."
In one of the workshops, someone asked, "Where is the book that goes with this class?" This question planted the seed, which gave birth to the book that you now hold in your hand: a book whose purpose is to get these healing teachings to all who are in need of them.

We return to our original question. We yearn for peace, quiet, yet exciting and joy-filled lives. So we wonder, can life be different? Is there a way off the drama dance floor? These teachings proclaim a resounding "Yes!"

Guidelines For Using This Book

It's not the surface work that is needed now... It's the deep work. We need to bring our dreams and visions down to earth and put them in our lives. In my country we can't just stagger around in our visions—the rattlesnake teaches us that. We need to be awake and pay attention to where we put our feet.
Native American Elder

This healing approach— *Three Turns of the Kaleidoscope*—is the "deep work." But wait! Put away your shovel and your work gloves and your serious frowned face and your brute force and all those ways you may have used over the years to make things happen. Those types of actions and attitudes are not needed and are truly ineffective here.

Instead, you are invited to slip into the comfortable clothes of soft breathing, of relaxed muscles, of eyes cast inward, and mind quiet.

As the Kaleidoscope turns, the Universal Healing Energy brings Light into deep crevices. Hidden there, vital information may be revealed in the terrain of who you are, on what is running inside you.

This book is divided into the stages of the Healing-The-Victim-Within journey, from a time of Innocence as a Healthy Natural Mammal, through Separation from our essential selves while living in Drama, to Initiation into a transformed way of being, and finally wending our way to Return to Wholeness. To illuminate, magnify, and clarify these stages, the reader will find references and stories of the author's healing journey of innocence, separation, initiation, and return in which Drama and victim-hood are transcended and Wholeness is re-membered.

Part I—Harnessing Cosmic Energies—begins with an overview of the whole healing process laid out on a diagram of three six-pointed stars nestled within each other. It continues with the chapter, "Why Triangles?" which covers the healing gifts of sacred geometry. A pictorial step-by-step overview precedes the in depth coverage of the first preparatory step: invoking the healing energy of six-pointed star.

Part II—Innocence—is a comprehensive discussion of the second preparatory step: Remembering our Healthy Natural Mammal.

Part III—Separation—is a thorough presentation of the third preparatory step: Choosing our Drama Dance experience.

Part IV—Initiation—contains the specific teachings for healing-the-Victim-within through the three kaleidoscopic turns. These teachings include the applications of sacred geometry, the hands-on energetic healings, the incisive questions and the transformational spiritual qualities (truth, forgiveness, self-love, wisdom, compassion and higher purpose). The power and wonder of this healing process resides in the energetic healing meditations and interventions as well as the applications of sacred geometry. Without them the questions may help our ordinary understanding of the Drama Dance. With them, the Drama Dance is transformed and the internalized victim is offered healing.

Part V—Return to Wholeness—brings us full circle to an awareness of who we are and how we can live our daily lives as whole beings.

Part VI—Resources—includes the how's and why's for answering the incisive questions, the personal stories of healing the drama, step-by-step instructions for the energetic healing techniques, the bibliography and a complete overview of the healing process.

Laid out in an orderly approach, the book guides you step by step. Just keep turning the pages and following the directions and you will complete three turns of the kaleidoscope bringing you a true vision of who you are.

Definitions

Compare the words in ALL CAPS with the standard dictionary definitions.

Words in this column are definitions specifically for *Three Turns of the Kaleidoscope*	Words in this column are standard definitions from Miriam-Webster Dictionary Tenth Edition
VICTIM: One that is acted on and adversely affected by an **internal** force or agent, usually one's feelings, thoughts and beliefs.	**Victim:** One who is acted on and usually adversely affected by an external force or agent. p. 1316
RESCUER: One who helps or takes care of another or oneself when such help or care is not needed and sometimes is actually harmful. Considers persons being helped as unable to help themselves.	**Rescuer:** One who frees from confinement or danger through prompt and/or vigorous action. p. 995
PERSECUTOR: One who harasses in a manner designed to injure, grieve or afflict self or other who has the means to defend self and does not. The VICTIM and PERSECUTOR cooperate in the Drama Dance, creating and perpetuating misery and shame for all.	**Persecutor:** One who harasses in a manner designed to injure, grieve, or afflict. p. 886
KALEIDOSCOPE: An imaginary toy-like instrument containing tiny particles of information and mirror-like reflections. When turned, different patterns emerge, providing a shift in awareness.	**Kaleidoscope:** A toy or instrument containing tiny colored particles and mirrors. When shaken or turned, different visual patterns are reflected off the mirrors. Adapted from p.637
RE-MEMBER: 1. To become aware of the many aspects or personalities or facets of our souls that may have been lost or hidden from our awareness. 2. To bring all the members of whom we are into one consciousness	**Remember:** to bring to mind or think of again p. 989
DRAMA DANCE: An internalization of oneself as Victim and subsequent misery-producing drama-like interactions	**Drama:** A state, situation, or series of events involving interesting or intense conflict of forces p.351

Definitions (con't)

Heal: to re-member oneself as whole and holy

Healer: one who serves as an instrument through which the universal healing energies flow and who provides energetic support and presence for self or other to heal.

Healing-The-Victim-Within: a multi-faceted process for healing an internalization of Victim and the ensuing Drama. This process is an intentional coming together of sacred geometry, energetic healing techniques, and incisive questions.

Human Energy System: subtle vibrations that power an individual human on all levels: physical, emotional, mental and spiritual. The vibrations form an integrated and interconnected grid that both carry and process complex information. This system is often described as fields of energy (aura), processing centers (charkas) and pathways (meridians). People can perceive these vibrations by seeing, hearing, feeling, smelling, tasting and knowing.

Chakras: processing centers that are concentrated matrixes of energy. In the East Indian Vedic tradition, the Sanskrit word means "wheels of light." Numbering in the hundreds these powerful vortices of light transform faster, more subtle energies into the more useable slower vibrations of matter in this earth plane as well as transform the denser earth energies into the uplifting and transcendent subtle energies.

Energy Fields: circles of energetic influence that emanate in an egg-shaped manner around and throughout living matter. The circles vary in strength, magnitude, frequencies, color, pattern and function. The energy fields of individual life forms, including humans, interweave and interact becoming a universal web of life.

Meridians: energetic flow lines that carry the vital life force throughout the human body, even to the nucleus of each cell.

Universal Healing Energies: cosmic forces that are subtle vibrations with the capacity to repair, restore, and enhance the well being of all life forms. Often associated with spiritual beings: God, Allah, Christ, Kwan Yin, Mother Mary and spiritual phenomena: Light, Warmth, Sacred Heart, Divine Love.

Pointers

USE the energetic healing techniques first, last and in between. When in doubt or stalled, choose one of the energetic healing technique described on pages 117-132.

AUGMENT the essence of these teachings through reading the personal stories, studying the diagrams and playsheets. The charts, diagrams, personal stories, and examples are especially helpful in clarifying and recognizing the three roles in the Drama Dance.

COMPLETE the playsheets in each chapter. Using colored pencils and rulers to draw the triangles creates an energetic internalization of the healing effects of the sacred geometry. Part One explores the questions—"Why triangles?" and "Why do we need to draw the triangles?"—asked by many when they encounter these teachings.

Diagram (opposite page): The entire healing process for *Three Turns of a Kaleidoscope* is laid out on three six-pointed stars. Nestled within each other, the stars depict a multidimensional and vibrant healing energy. The outermost and largest six-pointed star serves as a symbol for the cosmic template that harnesses powerful universal healing energies. Note the six spiritual qualities vibrating at the six outer points. On the middle star, the six small, outer triangles correspond to the six personal actions (three preparations and three turns) for healing the Victim within. The center star represents the cosmic template internalized in the core of our whole beings.

Part I: HARNESSING COSMIC ENERGIES

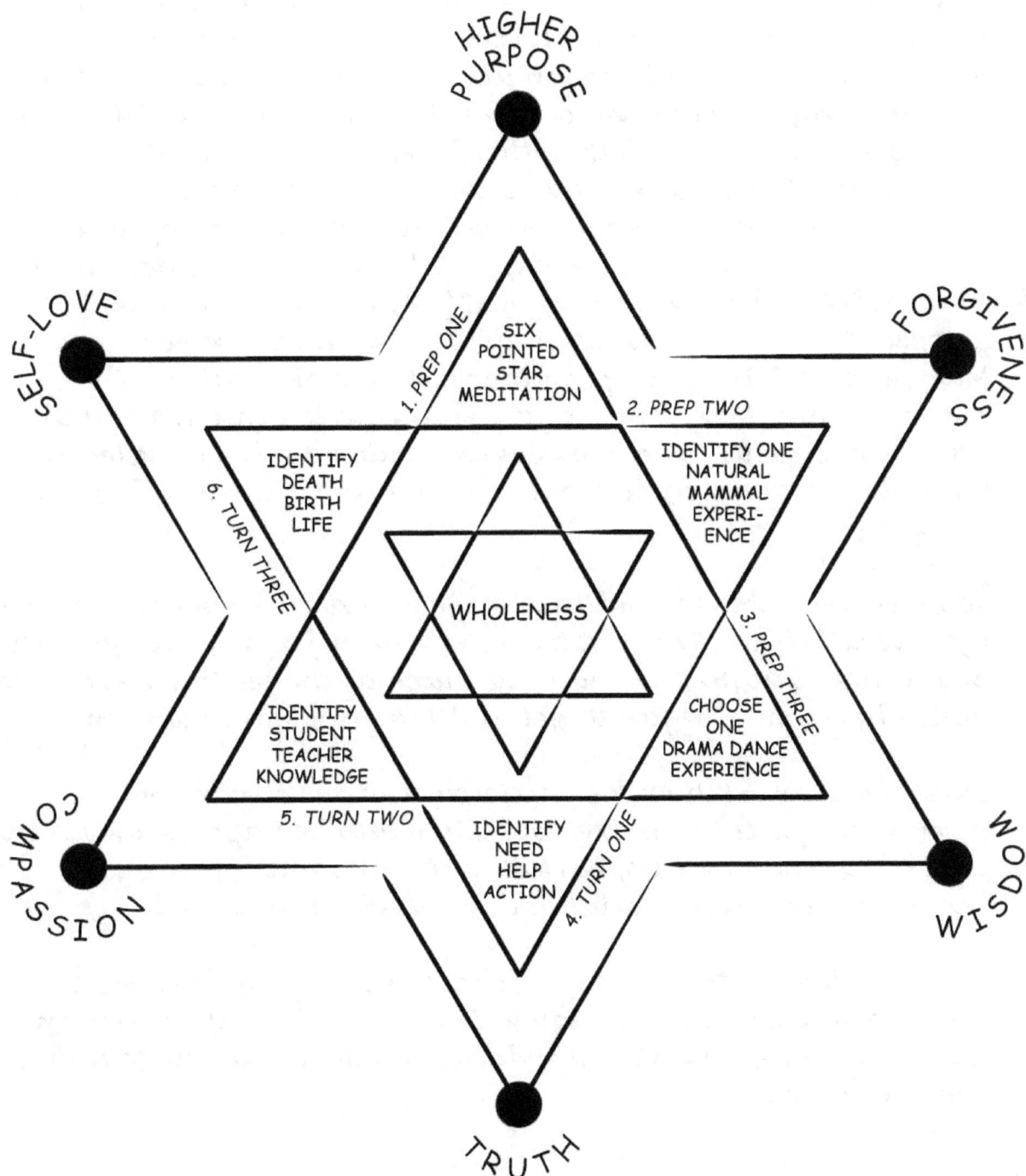

© 2008 Three Turns of a Kaleidoscope by Bonnie Johnson – Permission granted to duplicate for personal and educational purposes.

Memoirs

<u>Winter 2005 Delaware Beach</u> Colored pencils, graph paper, plastic compasses and rulers cover the kitchen table where Lois, Marty and I gather. Marty, as a child, had played with all this paraphernalia for hours on hours. She was relaxed and maybe a little bored by the afternoon activity. She easily twirled the compass around, creating circle after circle and triangle after triangle. Lois and I, on the other hand, held our compasses awkwardly. Our muscles were tense, our breathing labored, our brows were a farm acre of furrows. Our circles were lop-sided, our triangles crooked. Marty yawned; Lois threw up her hands and said: "Why are we doing this?" My hand cramped as I gripped the compass; I answered, "I really don't know except Mary said to." In developing the workshop on Healing-The-Victim-Within, Mary, the Magdalena gave the instructions to have participants use compasses and rulers to draw circles and triangles. We persevered, debating whether Mary was off base this time.

Soon we were able to hold the compass and make marks without hyperventilating. The first true circle drew yelps of wild joy! The emerging triangle stunned us as much as the setting sun on the ocean horizon. I began to get a glimmer of Mary's wisdom.

Later, in the workshops, as participants drew circles and triangles, something mysterious seemed to be happening within the bodies and brains of participants. Energetic openings, increased confidence, and a quiet satisfaction spread.

Mary invites you to cross the uncharted waters of drawing true circles and emerging triangles. It is worth the trip. Marty on the other shore, smiles and nods her head in welcome to us first-time explorers.

Why Triangles?

Sacred Geometry is the blueprint of Creation and the genesis of all form. It is an ancient science that explores and explains the energy patterns that create and unify all things and reveals the precise way that the energy of Creation organizes itself. On every scale, every natural pattern of growth or movement conforms inevitably to one or more geometric shapes.
Light Source[8]

Drawing on the knowledge of sacred geometry, the process for healing the Victim within intentionally uses shapes and numbers to bring in higher vibrational energies for healing and heightened awareness. The illustration of the three six-pointed stars nestled inside each other (page 17) is a graphic representation of this healing process. It clearly reveals a plethora of triangles. The outermost and largest six-pointed star serves as a symbol for the cosmic template that harnesses powerful universal healing energies. Emanating from the six points of the two largest and interwoven triangles are the spiritual qualities: truth, self-love, forgiveness, compassion, wisdom and higher purpose. The six smaller and outer triangles of the middle star correspond to the six personal actions (three preparations and three turns) for healing the Victim within. The center six-pointed star represents this cosmic template internalized in the core of our beings.

The triangle, first born of all geometric shapes, plays a major role, both as a foundation and as a portal. Why triangles? The following exploration of sacred geometry provides geometric and energetic underpinnings for the use of the triangle as a model of the Drama Dance <u>and</u> as a subtle yet powerful energetic form for healing.

Let's unwrap this geometric gift by examining it in three different sections:
   One, the characteristics and qualities of the triangular shape;
   Two, the meaning and significance of the number three in relationship
        to the whole; and
   Three, the cosmic influence and power of the six-pointed star.

---

8 www.sacred-geometry.com

The Characteristics and Qualities of Triangles

The ancients considered triangles to be the basic building blocks of the universe. From the long ago discovery of the triangle until today, wise builders have used this geometric form to provide structure and stability. In the world of energetic healing, the universe is perceived as subtle vibrational gridlines, which intersect to form geometric blueprints. Specifically, the triangle, which appears over and over in these universal patterns, is a vibrating portal through which copious energies can and do flow. By adding a healing intention, this geometric template becomes perfect for drawing in an abundance of healing energies.

A triangle can be described as a closed shape having three sides and three angles. A quick look at various constructions—sawhorses, swing sets, building buttresses—will reveal the presence of this geometric shape. In using geometry for building, the triangle was and is "...necessary to create self-supporting structures" which are rigid, strong and stable.[9]

In defining geometry as the "measurement of the earth" the ancients used the knowledge of the different geo-measurements to guide them as they built structures. They were aware that, through the shape of structures, they were connecting with and drawing on the universal energies.[10] In *Constructing the Universe*, Michael Schneider writes, "The triangle is a visually arresting shape and powerful symbol...(It) implies a message of wholeness...."[11]

The birth of an equilateral triangle is one of elegance, mysticism and distinction. Geometers do not use a free-hand sketch; they use an exact approach and precise qualities to create a triangle. This is how they do it: Using a compass and pencil, they select a center point and a length for the radius, and then they draw a circle. Next, they place the compass on any point on the circumference and draw a second circle. Looking at the diagram on the opposite page, we see two circles of the same radius and circumference. The inner edge of each circle intersects precisely with the center point of the other circle. A lens-shaped opening appears where the two

---

[9] Michael Schneider p.45
[10] Margaret Starbird p. 20
[11] Michael Schneider p. 41

Why Triangles? 21

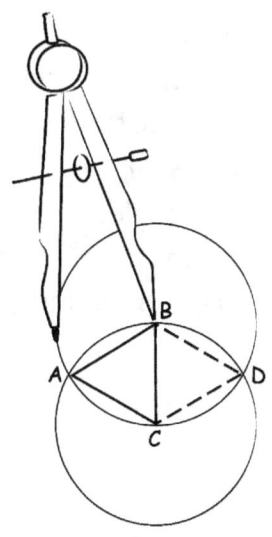

circles overlap. Using a ruler and pencil, the geometer draws lines from point **A** to point **B** to point **C**, creating a closed shape with three sides and three angles.

The triangle is the first shape that a geometer brings through this special opening. Known as the vesica piscis (which is Latin for "eye of the fish"), it is often likened to the birth canal of the Divine Mother. It is the portal through which structure is born. Sacred Geometry, with its intentional use of shapes to bring in higher vibrational energies, perceives the triangle to be "birthed from an unspeakable archetypal level into configuration." It is the first born which prepares the way for all other geometric forms. The triangle, therefore, is a blueprint or a template, which channels the universal energies to earthly and human arenas.[12]

Placing the Drama Dance on a triangle was a brilliant move by Stephen Karpman. Since the triangle is both a strong and stable form, it accurately mirrors those same qualities of the Drama Dance. The DD is so strong and so stable that it is like a self-perpetuating machine. It thrives on itself. This subtle vibrational form lends itself to increased energy flow, drawing us to it. In the Drama Triangle, like a gigantic tornado, we experience the feelings of being sucked into a chaotic and disturbing way of relating, and helpless to extract ourselves from the Drama.

On the human level, these disturbing energies are what persons experience after breaking free from being physically restrained against their will. With the breaking free, a person will often display chaotic behaviors: running in erratic circles; trembling, shaking and jerking of muscles; pounding heart; striking out and hitting; and angry screams and shouts. This is the bodily discharging of pent-up fight-or-flight energy.[13] Without an avenue for release, these trapped turbulent energies fuel the entrenchment of the Drama Dance.

---

12 Michael Schneider p. 43

13 Peter Levine Waking The Tiger pp. 19-21

In healing the Victim within, just as in the Drama Dance, the characteristics of the triangle (stability, strength, conduit for powerful and generous energies) are tapped. However, these energies are different from those that feed the Drama. These are healing energies that are the faster, subtler vibrational frequencies of restoration. Instead of chaotic and disturbing energies, calm and ordering energies flow through the healing triangles that are the first, second and third turns of the kaleidoscope, providing a counter-force that gently transcends the Drama. The essential self is restored and a holistic settling into one's skin occurs.

The Power of Three's

Geometry is the bridge between one and many.
Michael Schneider

The triangle's power which fuels and sustains the Drama Dance <u>and</u> restores and transforms the Victim within is not limited to its shape. This power also includes the energetic significance of the number three. Again, let's look to the wisdom of our ancestors.

Eighteenth century French novelist Honore` de Balzac writes, "Three is the formula of all creation" echoing the geometers' assertion of the triangle as harbinger of all geometric forms. In the creation of mammalian new life, we put together sperm, egg and the right environment. Schneider describes this as taking opposing poles (sperm and egg); adding a binding element (right environment) to bring forth a new whole (baby mammal). He continues: "We feel its correctness and express it through our words and images." [14]

For instance, we often talk about a whole by describing its three parts. We relate a story by telling beginning, middle and end. The three dimensions of length, width, and height define a particular space, like a board or poster. Our lives are lived through the lens of time: past, present, future. In telling you about my garden, I use the words: "I am getting ready to plant" or "Pretty soon the lilacs will be just right to cut and bring in the house for the last sweet aroma of the season" or "Everything in the garden is resting in its

---

[14] Michael Schneider p. 38-41

winter hibernation." These words reflect the planting cycle of sowing, harvesting and dormancy[15]

The idea of things, events, and processes coming in three's "emerge(s) from deep inside us... Three announces wholeness and completion through embracing syntheses." Often this bringing together of two opposites and a binding element creates something that is strengthening, invigorating and empowering. For example, take a rock, flint and dry leaves. Strike the flint against the rock to produce a spark that lands on the dry leaves and fire is produced. The spark-fire is a new resource that is stronger and more powerful than the three components alone. My favorite example is: mix together an artist, a medium such as clay, and a large dose of Inspiration to bring forth Art, a literal new creation that can continue to stir our aesthetic senses.[16]

In *Life After Death* Deepak Chopra notes that three requisites are involved in creating meaning in consciousness. From the teachings of the five thousand year old Vedic tradition in India, the three elements are 1) the observer, 2) the process of observing and 3) the thing observed. The "ancient sages hit upon a universal rule of consciousness, called three-in-one." Chopra asserts, "If you occupy any of these roles—seer, seen, or the process of seeing—you occupy them all." [17]

When a person (observer) notices (process of observing) herself (the thing observed) instantly there is this three-in-one state. An observer beholds an object through the process of observation. "Only in the unity of all three roles do we achieve our complete power as creators." Only when we observe ourselves doing the Drama Dance do we have the unity, therefore the consciousness to "achieve our complete power as creators" of our own life.

In healing the Victim within, each of the three healing triangles (Turn One, Two and Three) has three aspects. These three aspects in each triangle come together and create something new: an awareness, a perspective and a consciousness that powers a new way of relating to self and others.

---

15 Michael Schneider p. 38-41
16 Michael Schneider p. 38-41
17 Deepak Chopra p. 162

The Cosmic Influence of the Six-Pointed Star

The six-pointed star, as an energetic form, is both the foundation and apex of this healing process. The highest, fastest and subtlest healing energies flow through this form into the earth and human energy systems. It is a religious symbol as the Star of David or Seal of Solomon in the Jewish faith, the Mark of Vishnu in the Hindu spiritual path, and the Marian star in the Roman Catholic teachings. Nature reveals the template of the six-pointed star in snowflakes, frozen crystallized water, and quartz crystals. Many temples and cathedrals, including the Roslyn Chapel in Scotland, Notre Dame at Chartres in France, and Stonehenge in England, all share this geometric form in their design, function or structure.

Let's look at what sacred geometry and the ancients teach us about the six-pointed star. This form is constructed by interlacing two triangles: one pointing upward and one downward. The common space shared by both triangles is a hexagon with six equal sides and six equal angles.

Margaret Starbird in *Magdalene's Lost Legacy* informs us that the downward pointed triangle ▼ is "associated with Mother Goddess..." as well as being a "...prehistoric symbol for the ...womb of all life..." a representation of the Great Earth Mother. Seen as a sacred container and creative vessel.... this archetypal chalice is symbolic of the Eternal Feminine. Often described as the water triangle, we may be reminded of our first days swimming in the amniotic waters of our mother's womb.[18] In healing the Victim within, this symbolic cup is a container that receives energy. It is associated with the spiritual qualities of truth, forgiveness, and self-love and the frequencies of the throat chakra (see page 23).

The upward pointed triangle ▲ represents the procreative power of the Great Father or Father Sky or the Sun God. It is perceived to be the masculine or fire triangle that reminds us of the power of action and focus. On the body level, this triangle represents the male phallus, which powers the release of life-creating sperm upward into the receptive womb triangle.[19] In healing the Victim within this is a symbolic quality that sends energy. It is

---

[18] Starbird p. 10-12
[19] Starbird p. 10-12

associated with the qualities of wisdom, compassion and higher purpose and the energies of the brow chakra. (See pages 32-33).

Together the two triangles, ▲ and ▼, create the six-pointed star; it represents a uniting of the sacred feminine and the sacred masculine. Here, the receptive and active movements of energy merge. The ancients might say that it is the marriage of the sun god and earth goddess. In this marriage, the god and goddess become ONE. This is a sacred union that is likened to nirvana or bliss. All distinctions that separate have been transcended into the experience of ALL THAT IS.[20] The frequencies of the throat and brow merge into the oneness of the crown chakra. (See page 32).

This interwoven design serves as a template for creating physical constructions, such as temples, precisely to receive the cosmic energies and principles of the universe. In the earth planes, the six-pointed star is the archetypal template of the cosmic temple and represents the intimate union that brings peace, harmony, and well being to the community that surrounds a temple.[21]

The geometric configuration of the six-pointed star serves as a template for the healing meditation described on pages 30-31. In this meditation, we are building the archetypal template of the cosmic temple (universal energies) within our surrounding community, that is, within our human energy fields. Therefore, it serves as the template or temple for oneness that is experienced within us as peace, harmony and well being.

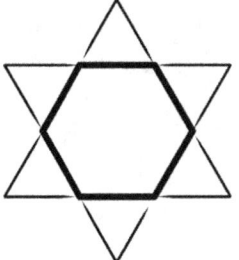

As noted earlier, in the world of energetic healing, the triangle has been and is a subtle vibrational form through which copious energies can and do flow. The common space shared by the interwoven triangles, ▲ and ▼, is a hexagon. The universal energies flowing through this hexagonal portal are exponentially greater than the flow through just one energetic triangle.[22] This greater force is the healing influence that powers the healing of the Victim within.

---

20 Starbird p. 10-12
21 Starbird p. 20
22 Nick Herbert p. 75 "Wave energy goes as amplitude squared. When you double a wave's amplitude, you quadruple its energy content."

When we examine the printed recording of vibrating frequencies, such as the electrical fluctuations of the human heart or vocal cords, we note wavy ups and downs. The most stable electrical fluctuations are recorded as the fewest cycles per second, with the lowest energy. These fluctuations are often referred to as slow or low frequencies. The fast or upper or subtle frequencies are less stable and thus more easily changed. This means that more energy is needed to effect a change in a slow, stable vibratory state than in a faster vacillating pulsation.

The energetic pattern of the Drama Dance depicts stable, slow fluctuations and is difficult to change. Through the six-pointed star, the fast and powerful healing energies are harnessed for transforming this stable, often entrenched pattern.

Summary

The triangular-shaped models of the Drama Dance and of healing the Victim within convey ancient knowledge and mystery regarding the power of triangles, the number three and the star hexagram. The strength of the energies flowing through these models attests to the powerful forces that keep us in the Drama and that are needed to release us from the Drama. The coming together of two triangles in the star hexagram harnesses the incredible energies that can and do heal the Victim within.

A Brief Overview
Three Turns of a Kaleidoscope: Healing Victim Within

This pictorial overview provides a quick glance at the entire healing-the-victim-within process. First read this overview, then the in-depth descriptions of the process in the following chapters. In addition, use this overview as a cue card for prompting the sequence.

PREP ONE:
Invoking the healing energy of six-pointed star

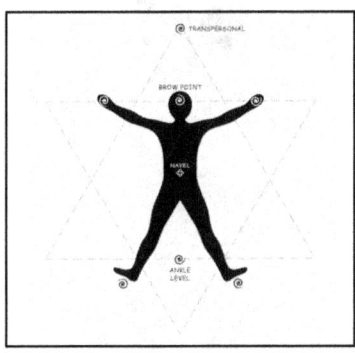

PREP TWO:
Recall one Natural Mammal experience in your life.

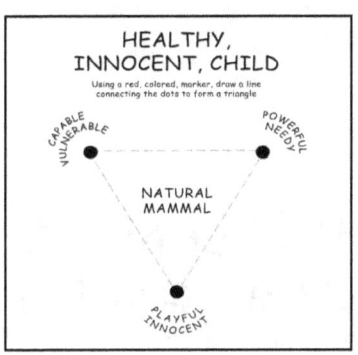

PREP THREE:
Choose one Drama Dance experience in your life.

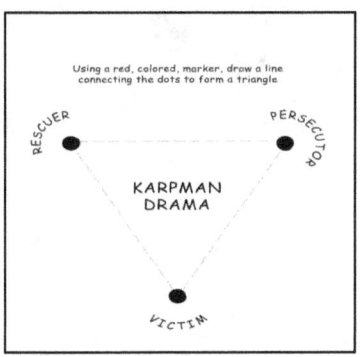

FIRST TURN:
Use your Drama experience: to Identify the Need, the Help and the Action

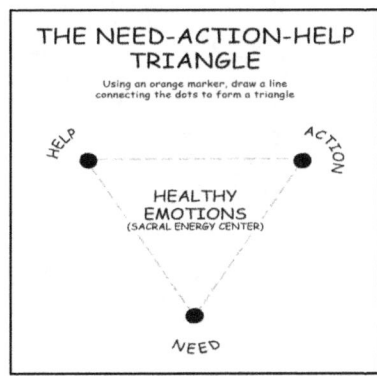

SECOND TURN:
In your Drama Dance, Identify the Student, the Teacher and Discover the Knowledge.

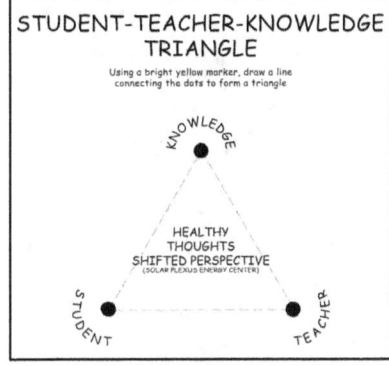

THIRD TURN:
In your Drama Dance, Identify the Death, the Birth, and then Reap the Living

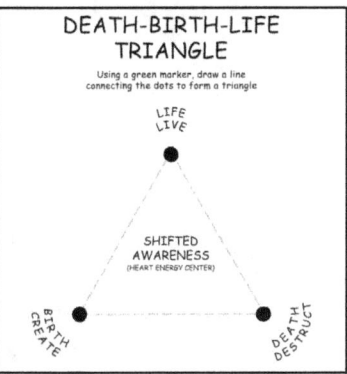

Now Celebrate!

© 2008 Three Turns of a Kaleidoscope by Bonnie Johnson – Permission granted to duplicate for personal and educational purposes.

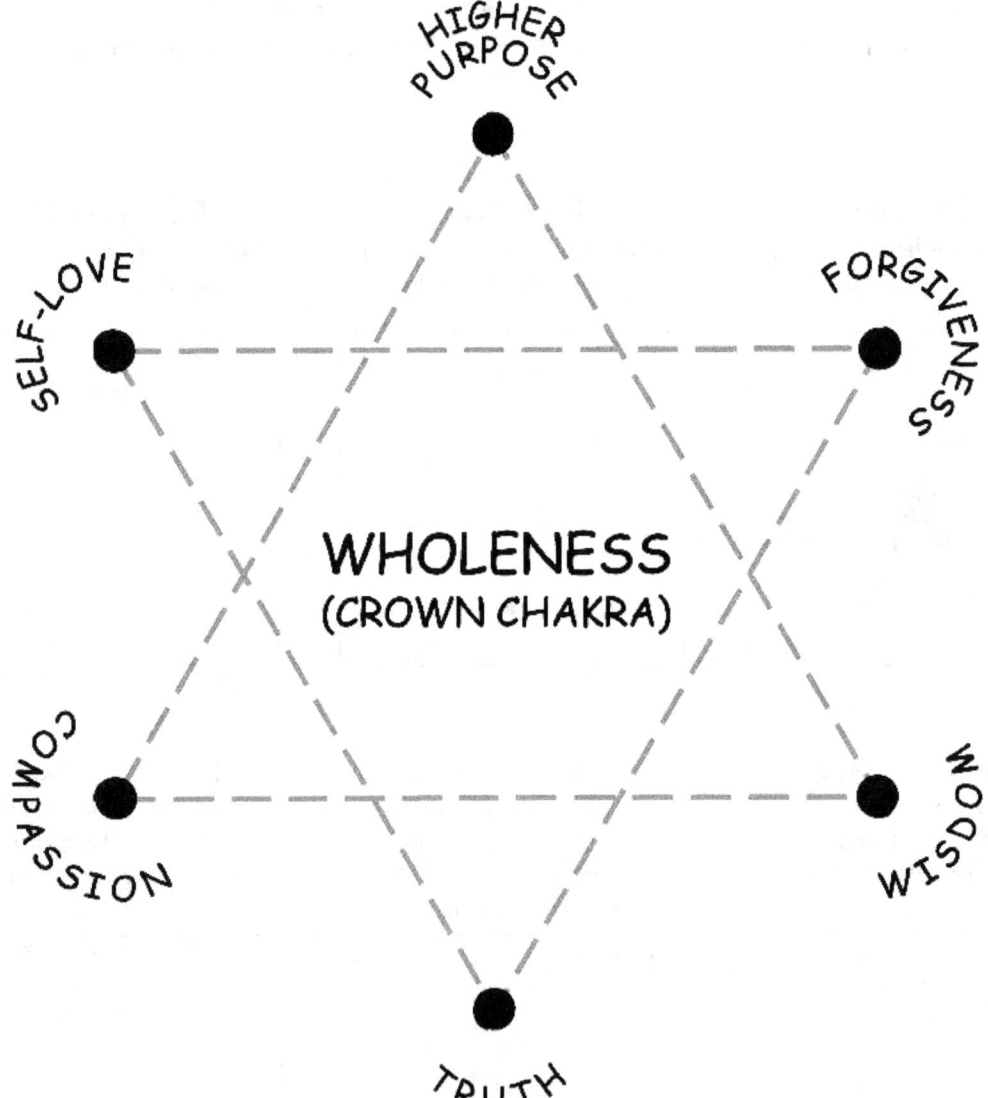

Prep One:
Accessing the Healing Energies

> **PREP ONE**
> ⚘ Complete or trace the drawings of the Six-Pointed Star with a marker.
>
> ⚘ Do the Six-Pointed Star Meditation

We begin healing the Victim within by using the energetic template of the six-pointed star to access the star's six spiritual qualities and to activate its energetic flow lines within our human energy systems.

The restorative vibrations—necessary for healing the Victim within—are subtle spiritual energies, which may be experienced as the qualities of self-love, forgiveness, truth, compassion, wisdom, and higher purpose. Through the light of these qualities, the Drama Dance is examined, transformed and transcended.

Take a moment now to complete the diagram of the six-pointed star on the opposite page. Tracing along the dotted lines creates healing connections in our memories, bodies and brains, which activates the spiritual energies of the six qualities laid out on star. Use the color violet to help blend the six qualities into the vibration of wholeness within your energy system.

The human energy system is made up of subtle vibrations that power an individual human on all levels: physical, emotional, mental and spiritual. The vibrations form an integrated and interconnected grid that carry and process complex information. Humans and other mammals detect these fluctuating vibrations by seeing, hearing, feeling, smelling, tasting and knowing and perceive them as colors, sounds, textures, temperatures, movement and images.

The human energy system is rich with the concentrated matrixes of energy that are called chakras in the East Indian Vedic tradition.[23] For this first preparatory step, we will focus on eight out of the hundred or more of these powerful vortices of light. The eight chakras are: transpersonal, crown, brow, throat, navel, ankle level, palms and feet.

---

23 Charles Leadbetter

The Six-Pointed Star Meditation

In the six-pointed star meditation, we trace the six-pointed star within our human energy systems. We access a supportive geometric structure and a powerful and transformational gateway as well as activate the six spiritual qualities of truth, self-love, forgiveness, compassion, wisdom and higher purpose. Received as guidance directly from the invisible being who identified herself as Mary, the Magdalena, this healing practice may also be repeated whenever additional energetic support is needed.

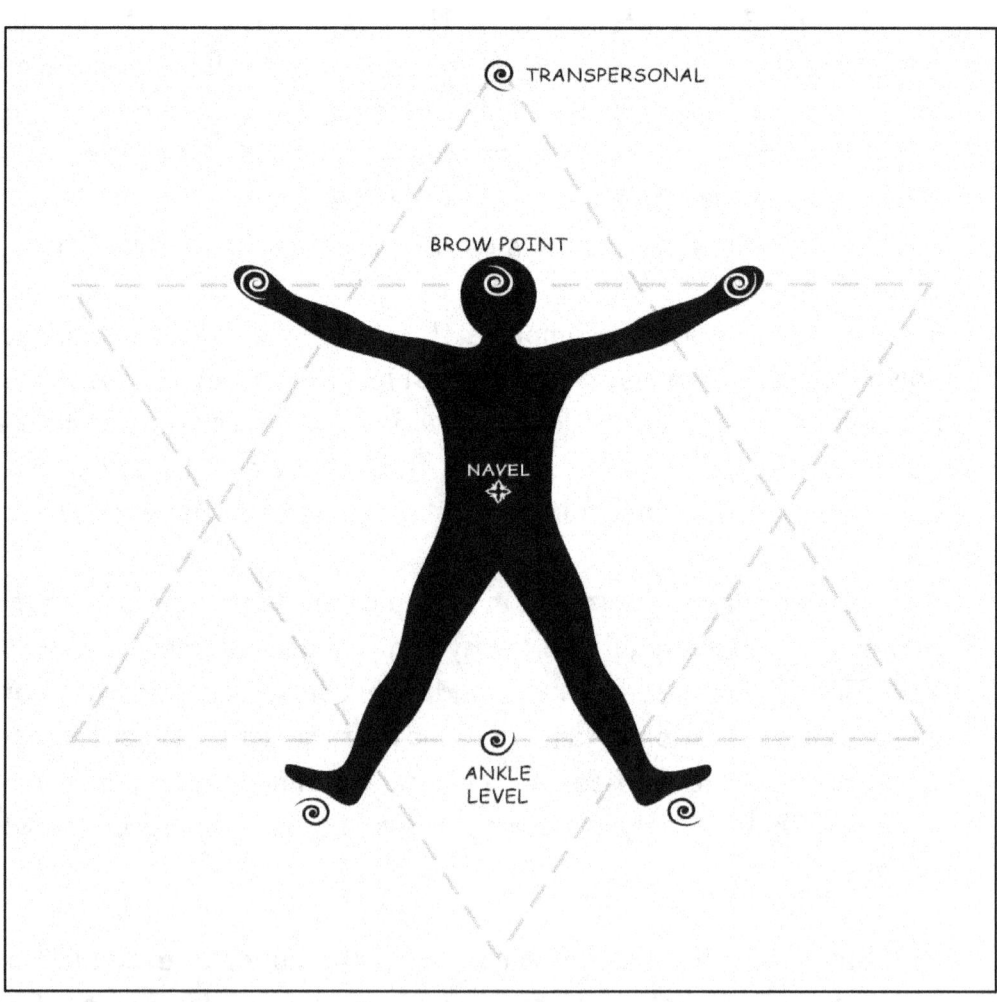

Instructions: Locate the chakras or energy centers on the diagram and on yourself: the palms of the hands, the soles of the feet, the brow – front and back, the chakra at the level of the ankles, the transpersonal and the navel. Notice the configuration of the six-pointed star is within the human energy system that extends about three feet beyond the physical body.

Trace the star in your human energy system with the following directions as a guide.

© 2008 Three Turns of a Kaleidoscope by Bonnie Johnson – Permission granted to duplicate for personal and educational purposes.

Six-Pointed Star Meditation

1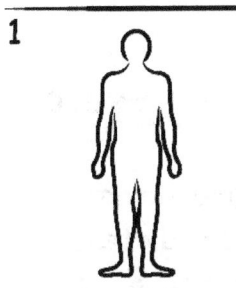

Prepare yourself for meditation by creating a space with as few distractions as possible. Sit or stand in a way that is physically comfortable for you. Let your attention move to your mid-chest. Quietly, observe yourself, breathing in and breathing out. No need to change your breathing. Just notice your breathing for a few minutes.

2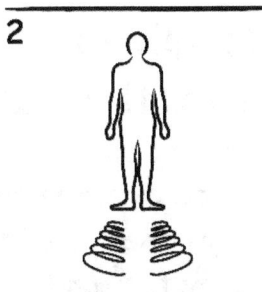

Gently, move your attention to the bottom of your feet. Become aware of the soles of your feet. Notice or imagine the energy centers at the bottom of your feet. Imagine that these moving vortexes of energy begin to activate, becoming stronger and stronger. Soon, you may notice the spinning flow reaching, from the soles of your feet, down into and resonating with the earth energies.

3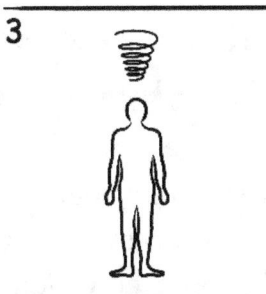

Slowly, move your attention to a spot about 18 inches above your head, letting your attention remain on this spot, known as the transpersonal energy center. Become aware of this energy center as a vortex of energy. Notice as it begins to activate, becoming stronger and stronger, flowing upward to the sun and resonating with the sun energies.

4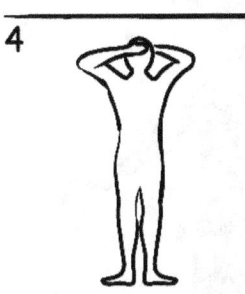

Place one hand on your brow, and the other hand on the back of your head. Allow life's healing energies to come through your hands and into your brow energy centers, front and back. Let yourself observe the brow energies for a minute.

5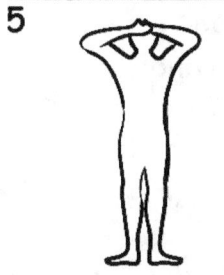

Slowly bring your rear hand from the back of your head to the front, putting it over the other hand so both hands cover the brow. Gently allow your hands to separate and move horizontally as far away from the midline of your body as possible.

6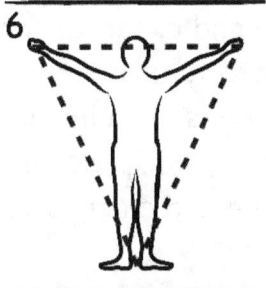

Your hands, following a horizontal energetic line, will be completely out to your sides and level with your brow. Then, pointing your hands down toward the ground, trace the energetic lines, toward the space between and beyond your feet. This forms the first energetic triangle.

7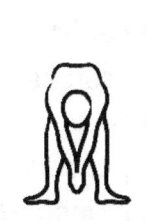

Place both hands into the space between your ankles, allowing the healing energies to come through your hands and into this space that is also an energy center. Gently allow your hands to separate and move horizontally.

8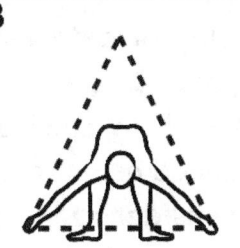

With your hands out as far away from your feet as possible, move your hands diagonally upward toward the ceiling/sun, meeting at a point over your head. You have traced the lines that form the second energetic triangle.

9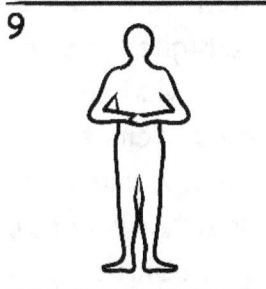

Move both hands to the navel, allowing the healing energies to come through your hands and into this powerful energy vortex. Rest in this awareness.

© 2008 Three Turns of a Kaleidoscope by Bonnie Johnson – Permission granted to duplicate for personal and educational purposes.

The Star's Six Spiritual Qualities through the Eyes of the Human Energy System

The six spiritual qualities are associated with the crown, brow and throat chakras, The crown chakra is located at the top of the head and radiates upward in an ever-widening cone of very fast and very subtle energies. It processes the energetic information that generates or brings into existence the experience of Wholeness. Here all the diverging qualities find peace; here the opposites melt into each other and become indistinguishable. There is no longer an up and a down or a back and a forward or a good and a bad. Here the energetic information is ALL. In the six-pointed star the intersecting of male and female, down and up, inner and outer, internal and external come together and cooperate to bring about something brand new which is lived in the crown chakra. Here, the past, present and future disappear and emerge as the eternal now.

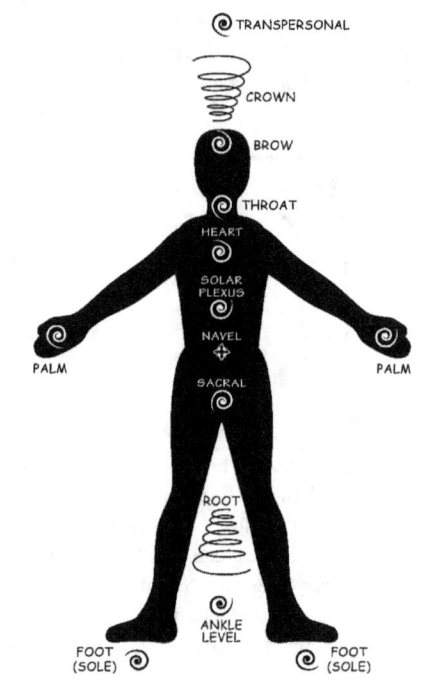

The triangle of Compassion-Wisdom-Higher Purpose is associated with the energy of the sixth or brow energy center, located at the level of the forehead and the back of the head directly behind the forehead. This chakra processes energetic information that generates or brings into existence higher (faster) vibrational manifestations including the qualities of compassion, wisdom and higher purpose. It also is related to expressions of extraordinary emotions, such as divine love, spiritual ecstasy, and bliss. Extraordinary emotions are experienced as uplifting, transforming and transcendent. The brow chakra is considered the locus of intuition, insight, and psychic abilities as well as telepathic rapport. Through the energies of the sixth chakra, we are able to see color and images of energy, hear guidance, and smell aromas of subtle frequencies.

The sound of rushing water is the frequency of a vibrant and active brow chakra. Sitting beside a stream that rushes down a mountain is a good way to activate the brow chakra energies and to seek spiritual guidance and insight.

The energies of the fifth or throat chakra support and power the triangle of Truth-Self Love-Forgiveness. The throat chakra is located at the cervical spine (neck) and the physical throat. It processes the energetic information that generates or brings into existence higher (faster) vibrational manifestations including the qualities or expressions of truth, self-love and forgiveness. Other qualities or expressions are: inspirational music, transformative ideas, living in accord with your life purpose, speaking words that are authentic as well as loving, gentle, incisive.

Wind blowing through the trees creates the same sound vibration as the throat chakra. Listen to the message in the wind. Hear the oscillations that resonate within you. Allow these vibrations to attune, activate and balance your throat energies.

Review and Summary of Prep One

Three Turns of a Kaleidoscope: Healing The Victim Within

In this first preparatory step, we accessed the star's spiritual energies by
1. Tracing the diagram of the six-pointed star, and
2. Doing the six-pointed star meditation.

In Parts IV and VI, three other ways for activating these energies are described:
3. Asking for the help of the qualities,
4. Studying and applying the meaning and knowledge of the qualities, and
5. Employing the healing technique: Chakra Correspondence.

Next, in Part II: Innocence, we enter into the realm of the healthy natural mammal, taking the second preparatory step in healing the Victim within.

NOTES:

Part II: INNOCENCE

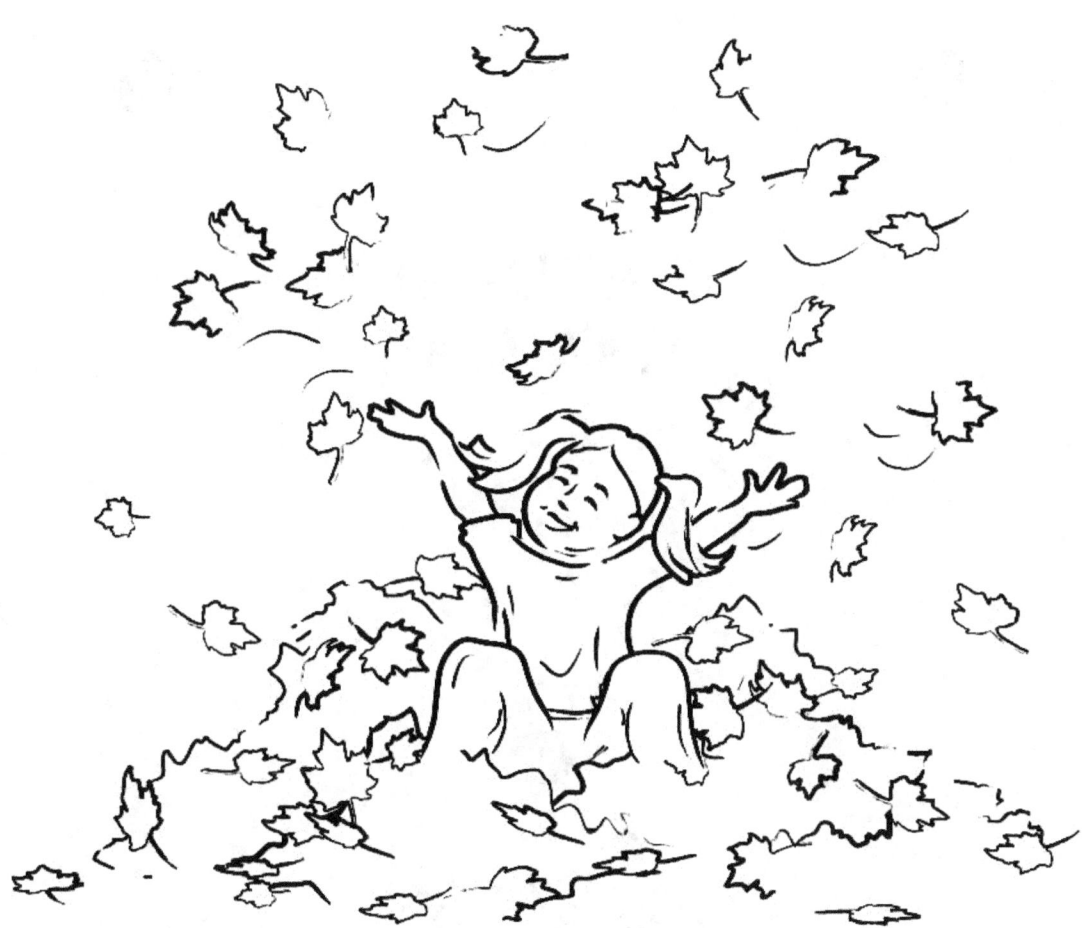

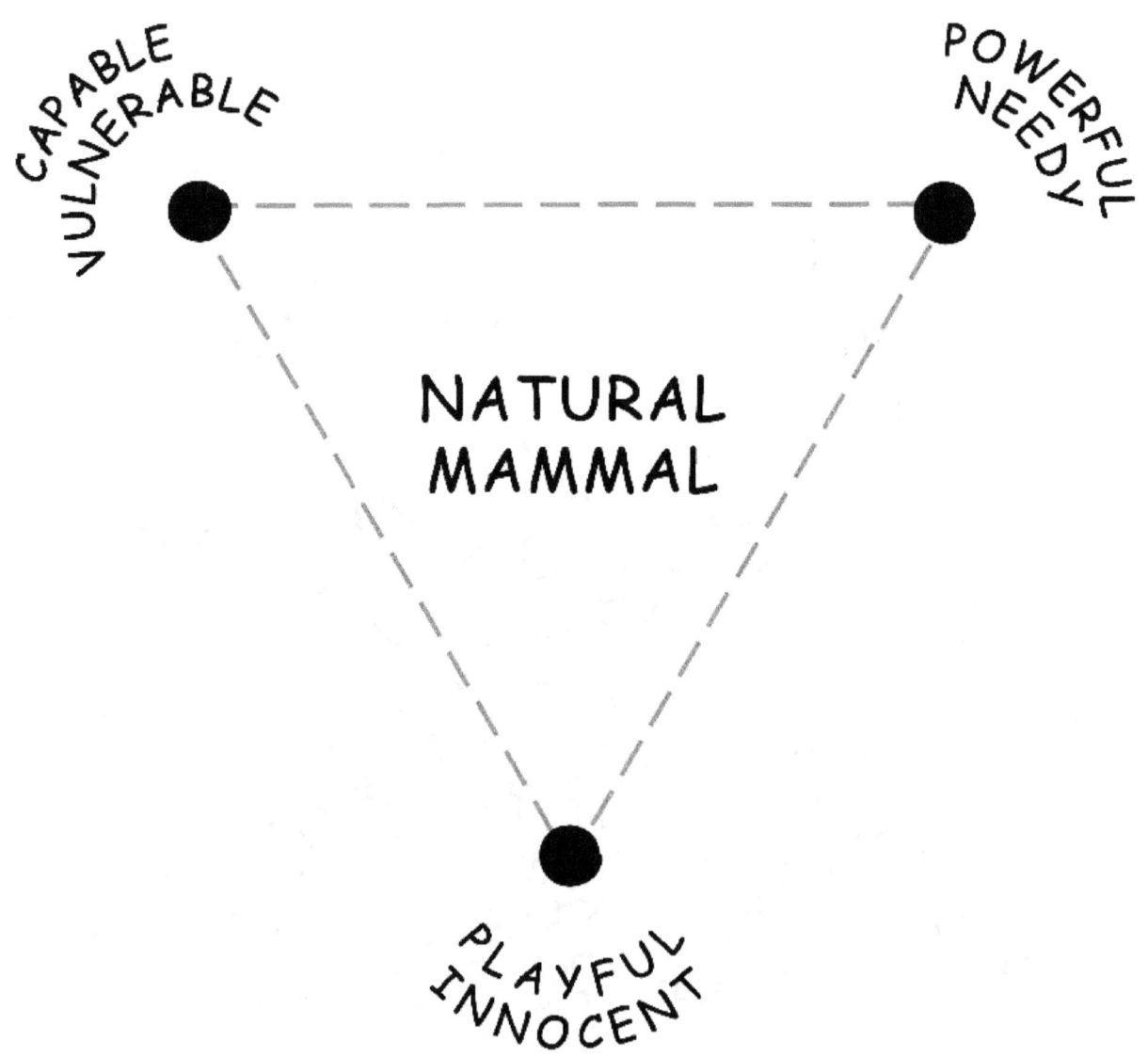

Prep Two: Recalling the Natural Mammal

> **PREP TWO**
>
> ⤻ Complete the drawing of the Natural Mammal triangle.
>
> ⤻ Identify one Natural Mammal experience in own life. Briefly share with a trusted person. This could be with oneself verbally or symbolically (writing, painting, dancing, sculpting...).

In Prep Two, we continue to prepare for the *Three Turns of the Kaleidoscope* (that helps us to heal the Victim within) by taking a moment to 1. Complete the Natural Mammal triangle. The completion of this triangle creates healing connections within our memories, bodies and brains. For this triangle, we use the color red to strengthen the vibration of red in our human energy systems and aid in healing the wounds related to trust, safety, security, survival and vitality.

Notice that the Natural Mammal triangle has two qualities for each of the three points of the triangle. The two qualities are not synonymous; instead they are poles apart and depict a correspondence that hints at a healthy balance. The natural infant mammal is both playful and innocent, both capable and vulnerable, both powerful and needy. As we observe natural mammals in action, we see them quickly switch and shift from powerful to needy, from playful to innocent, from vulnerable to capable.

After completing the triangle, we next 2. Identify a Natural Mammal experience in our own life. Teacher, activist and author, Parker Palmer encourages us to share "...childhood stories that contain clues about who we were before forces within and around us began to deform our sense of true self."[24] In the following, I share my first memory as an innocent, playful, and capable child.

Memoirs *October 1948 Lowell, Massachusetts*

The air is cooling and the curling maple leaves cover the side yard beside the four-story, clapboard home of my growing-up years. Although the house has eight large rooms, my siblings, parents and maternal grandparents and I fill every room with

---

[24] Parker Palmer p.81

barely enough space for the numerous cats, dogs, hamsters and fish. Having time alone or my own personal space is a rare treat. Summers, my favorite season, are spent in a rough cabin overlooking a New Hampshire lake. Here, plenty of alone time and more than enough personal space are available in the acres of woods where I roam.

Each September, we return to Lowell where my father operates his service station, where we attend school and church; where we play hide-and-go-seek in the yard and climb the "monkey bars" in the city field across the street. .

On this crisp October day, a neighbor girl and I gather the fallen leaves into a gigantic mound. Sitting down into the pile of leaves, my three-year-old self throws the red, orange and yellow leaves over my head. My arms stretch high above my head, forming a deep V. My head tips to the sky as the leaves rain down. I laugh and laugh and laugh, with each fresh shower of multi-colored leaves.

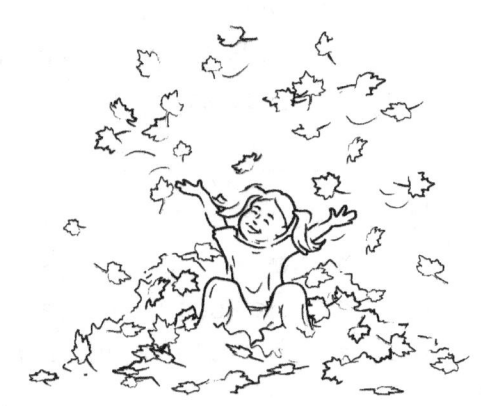

Meet Your Healthy Natural Mammal

What is your first memory of yourself as the innocent, playful, capable, vulnerable, powerful and needy child? You may need to dig deep to discover this child. Often many of us have had such abusive or neglected childhoods that this awareness is covered with too many layers of sh-t! Be patient, she or he is there in you and in your memory. Be assured by physician Charles Whitfield's word's: "No matter how distant, evasive, or alien it may seem to be, we each have a 'Child Within' – the part of us that is ultimately alive, energetic, creative and fulfilled."[25] Go find her or him!

---

25 Charles Whitfield p.9

Suggestions for uncovering and recalling:

- Watch for this child in any playful interactions in the present. Follow her or him back to your childhood.

- Draw a picture of the child with your non-dominant hand.

- Make up a story of this child: "Once upon a time in a small town, there lived a child ……"

- Look through photos of yourself as an infant or toddler.

- Take a clump of play dough and craft an image.

- Watch small children or animals (kittens are my favorite) as they play.

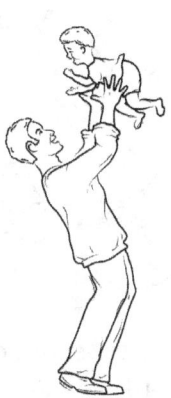

- Ask your older sibling, your great aunt, grandparent, or beloved family friend, what they remember about you as an infant or toddler. At age 25, Roger met his birth family for the first time in 24 years. One birth brother—15 years older—told Roger this story: " I remember you when you were a baby. I remember throwing you up in the air and catching you in my arms. We both laughed each time you flew into the air and sailed safely back into my arms."

- Experience hypnotherapy, shamanic journeying, hands-on energetic healing or art therapy as a way of accessing this essential aspect of you.

Once you have un-covered and re-membered a memory of yourself as the innocent, playful, capable, vulnerable, powerful and needy child, take the time to briefly share with a trusted person. This could be verbally or symbolically (writing, painting, dancing, sculpting) with your self or someone else or even a loved animal.

Most important is the knowledge that this is the healthy natural mammal—alive, energetic, creative and fulfilled—and through healing, the "child within" can be strong and alive in you and your present life.

Snapshots of the Natural Mammal

Fascination with body parts or specks of nothing captures the infant mammal's undivided attention for a millennium of now. Open mouths suck on paws, tails, toes, clothes; laughter fills the surrounding spaces; leaping joy sparks. Put two infant mammals of any species together and a sprawling play erupts: rolling, tickling, chasing, hiding, enticing, lapping, risking, adventuring, taking apart, tossing up into the air, and being that is pure glee. All mammals share these characteristics and experiences, including young children, tiger cubs and puppies. Scientist author, Joseph Pearce asserts that "...play absorbs the majority of a young child's life ...and is an incredibly varied and rich activity.... Playing is the natural way for all mammals to grow, explore, and mature...". [26]

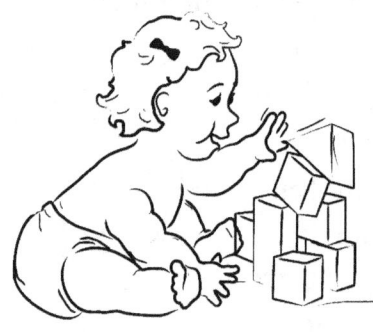

"A fat-legged toddler whoops with joy when she discovers she can knock over her tower of blocks. She is compelled to do it again and again, and each time the delight is undiminished," describes psychotherapist and guided imagery guru Belleruth Naparstek who adds that this experience is the toddler's teacher and the lesson is: "She is a prime mover; she can make things happen."[27] When an unknown person enters the toddler's space her joy turns to concern. Immediately, she looks around for a known caregiver. Spotting the caregiver, she rapidly crawls toward safety and away from perceived danger.

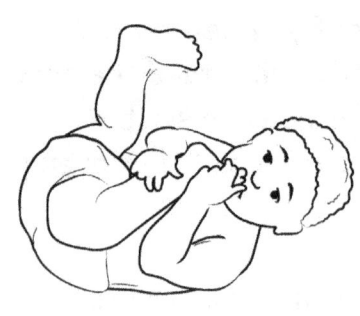

Six-month-old Maurice discovers his toe: he reaches out toward the toe, grasps it and brings it right to his mouth—takes it in—and fully experiences this other world known to observers as "his toe." But he does not do this as an objective researcher. He is fully engaged, playful, smiling, laughing, and sometimes, seriously focused. His self and his toe are fully present with each

---

26 Pearce page.141

27 Belleruth Naparstek p.39

other. The natural mammal "reaches out to the world, grasps pieces of it, takes them in and experiences them." [28]

This afternoon, as I meander down the sun-decorated, white-as-snow beach, two dogs streak down the steps and across the sand. Their entire bodies are smiles—unmistakably alive. They jump, wiggle, shake, roll, and nip at each other as if tasting pure delight.

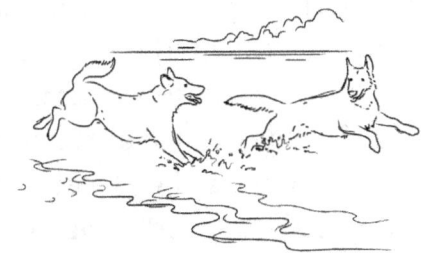

Four-year old Josephine wiggles as her father lowers her into the lake. Her arms and legs move quickly as she flops her body straight out. With her father's supporting hands under her abdomen, her awkward efforts propel her forward. She grins and shouts to her father: "I can swim, Daddy, I can swim!"

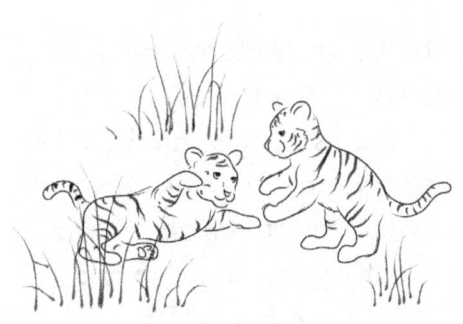

In the movie, *The Two Brothers*, the tiger cubs, Kumal and Sangha display natural mammal living with charm. Their deep innocent eyes draw in the viewer. Their free abandonment to play—rolling, licking, scuffing, jumping into the air after whiffs of wind, chasing each other through tall grasses, over rocks and debris, through their mother's legs—pull at that place in each of us that remembers our true mammal nature.

In another scene, tiger cub Kumal investigates a strange, fast-moving badger. The badger, not too keen on being bothered, turns and attacks. Kumal's curiosity has led him to unearth danger, and the big-eyed innocent, Kumal runs up a tree, searching for protection and crying out for help. His brother Sangha comes to his aid by scaring off the badger and encouraging Kumal who finally comes down from the tree and reaches the safe haven of his mother.

The natural infant mammal does not know the dangers that can hurt and kill. Pearce writes that "...Beneath all the studies and comments about animal and child play runs a central ...thread: **Play serves survival.**" (*bold added*)[29]

---

28 Starhawk p.54
29 Joseph Chilton Pearce p.141

Through play, the child, like all mammals, learns skills, awareness and behaviors that are transferred into the real world where danger lurks. Pearce notes that through play, the child learns the skills to indeed survive. Until that happens, the"...parents must assume responsibility for the child's survival." It is at the survival level that we witness the vulnerable and needy aspects of the natural mammal: the cries to be fed and the turning toward the safe older mammal for protection. Until the child has those skills, the adult protects and ensures the survival of the child. The vulnerability of the child is safeguarded. The needs—for the child is truly needy—are provided by the adult. Without the protection and provision of care, the child is hurt, or worse dies. Both trauma and dying may occur physically, emotionally, mentally, and spiritually.

When three-year-old Bonnie, tiger cub Kumal, Naparstek's toddler, four year-old Josephine and six- month-old Maurice act in ways that make something happen (full of power), they are fueling the awareness of themselves as capable. For children, especially four and under, the acting which makes something happen is related to play or reaching safety. When Naparstek's toddler saw a stranger enter the room and experienced "stranger anxiety," she looked around for a known caregiver. When she spotted the caregiver, she rapidly moved toward the caregiver and away from the stranger. All of these actions—seeing and recognizing a stranger, locating safe person and moving toward safe person—contribute to the child knowing herself as capable (able to) and powerful (affecting change in self, others and environment). Likewise, Kumal acted out of his vulnerability and need as he ran up the tree for protection. He learned that he was able to run from harm. When Jill and Sam's daughter Sarai was four years old, she spent an evening capturing lightning bugs in her cupped hands and watched them glow. The next morning, with her hands still filled with the glowing memory, Sarai reached out and cupped a bee that promptly stung her. In that simple encounter, her innocence was challenged. For the innocent mammal will just as soon play with a bee as a lightning bug. However, her survival required learning to tell the difference between the harmless and the harmful. As the older mammals in Sarai's life, Jill and Sam cared for her bite, soothed her feelings and gave her information about identifying safe lightning bugs.

Survival: a Celebration

Pearce writes that we have grim and gray ideas about survival. He suggests that survival is really about "victory of life over death." Survival is a celebration.[30]

In 2004, I was in a car accident in which a large truck "T-boned" into the driver's side of the car I was driving. In the nano-seconds before impact, I calmly thought, "So this is how I am going to die." After the impact, covered with glass, I kept touching my own body and saying, "I'm breathing. I'm breathing. I am still alive in my body." I experienced aliveness that was nothing less than euphoric. My whole body began trembling. The surge of adrenaline was at work. This surge signals that we are still alive; we have survived, and we do indeed celebrate our aliveness. We twirl and dance with the joy of still breathing.

"To be human, is to be born into a dance in which every animate and inanimate, visible or invisible being is dancing. Every step of this dance is printed in light; its energy is adoration, its rhythm is praise."[31] Watch an infant, in and out of utero and you will witness this dance. Travel back to your days inside your mother's womb and re-experience the dance-like movements of yourself. For our infant-selves know the flowing dance of this universe and participate with joy, play, and movement.

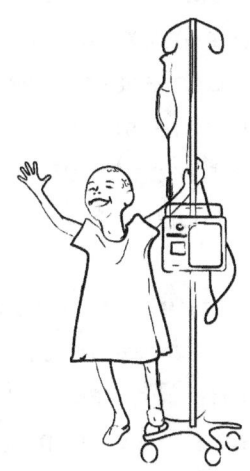

Though we grow up out of this infancy, the memory lingers. Six-year-old Obadiah rides the intravenous pole that carries the bags of fluid and the machine that distributes the fluids into his veins. Earlier in the morning, Obadiah felt so bad with pain in his hips and overtaking nausea that he laid motionless in bed. His body shows every rib, skin absent of fat, slight murmurs of hair left on his head. Feeling enough better, he now rides the hospital halls, looking for mischief – a gigantic grin covering his face. This is the natural mammal – let

---

30 Joseph Chilton Pearce p.141
31 Andrew Harvey p.26-27

loose for a few moments before the disturbances send him back to bed. "Play is its own reality experience, a state in which survival is always successful, where life always wins over death."[32] Obadiah rides that intravenous pole, celebrating the present moment in which he experiences himself alive and vibrant enough to play. He is not afraid to live fully, in spite of the many prior moments when he was literally close to death.

The psychotherapy literature abounds in descriptions of the healthy natural mammal that survives in the adult. Many names are given from "Child Within" to "Real Self, True Self, Inner Child, Divine Child, Higher Self, Deepest Self, and Inner Core." I add Essence, Essential Self, and Unchanging Self. The descriptions of this Essence are beautiful and inspiring as well as matching those of the natural mammal. Here is a sampling: "...the part of us that is ultimately alive, energetic, creative and fulfilled." "...who we are when we feel the most authentic." "... expressive, assertive, and creative.... It needs to play and have fun...it is vulnerable...open...trusting...surrenders itself to others and ultimately to the universe...yet is powerful...." [33]

The Natural Mammal through the Eyes of the Human Energy System

Let's describe this healthy child using another model: the human energy system. As described earlier, this system is made up of subtle vibrations that form an integrated and interconnected grid. This energetic grid carries and processes complex information. Recall that the human energy system is rich with concentrated matrixes of energy. The six-pointed star introduced the transpersonal, crown, brow, throat, palms, feet and ankle level energy centers. The natural mammal and the drama dance, respectively, are reflections of the healthy and distorted root chakra. The three turns of the kaleidoscope incorporate the crown, brow, throat, heart, solar plexus, and sacral chakras.

As natural mammals, we focus on the root energy center, so named because its energy connects us, grounds and roots us to the energies of the planet earth. The earth has a powerful electro-magnetic field that feeds and nourishes us continuously. When this root chakra is healthy, we experience

---

[32] Joseph Chilton Pearce p.142
[33] Charles L Whitfield p.9 & 10

ourselves as strong, protected, plugged-in, safe, secure, alive, vital, and with a sure trust in our own abilities, in our older caregivers and in our environment.

Pharmacist/shaman Connie Graud declares "All infants experience relatively unimpeded access to the vital energy that sustains them... Children live in this flow as long as their vital needs are met, their natural expressions are accepted, and they are loved, respected, cared for and are protected from danger, pain and trauma."[34]

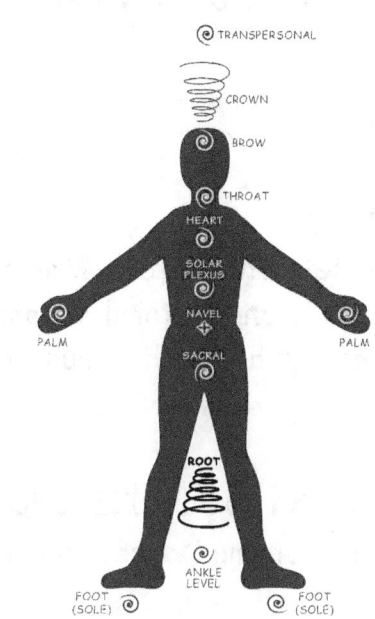

The root chakra energy is the base that lays the foundation for knowing ourselves as powerful. As children, this sense of trust and safety may not have been tested, so we remain innocent of potential dangers. As soon as Kumal, the tiger cub, encountered danger in the form of the aggressive badger, he sought help and ran up a tree. (A true metaphor for connection and protection in the guise of the earth!) Four-year-old Sarai encountered harm with the sting of a bee and received help and protection from her parents. With life's trauma (big or small), the root chakra encodes messages that help us to detect and avoid danger. In other words, these messages help us to survive: this is the job of the root chakra.

Recall what Pearce asserted: Survival is really about "victory of life over death." Survival is a celebration. Celebrations are declarations that we are still alive. We touch our bodies with the wonder that we still exist and we feel the joy of breathing, the joy of dancing.

---

[34] Connie Grauds and Doug Childers p.23

Review and Summary of Prep Two

Three Turns of a Kaleidoscope: Healing the Victim Within

PREP ONE
  Do the Six-Pointed Star Meditation.

PREP TWO
1. Complete the Natural Mammal Triangle drawing.
2. Identify one Natural Mammal Triangle experience in your own life. Briefly share with a trusted person.

Turn next to Part III: Separation and the third preparatory step: choosing a Drama Dance Experience.

NOTES:

Part III: SEPARATION

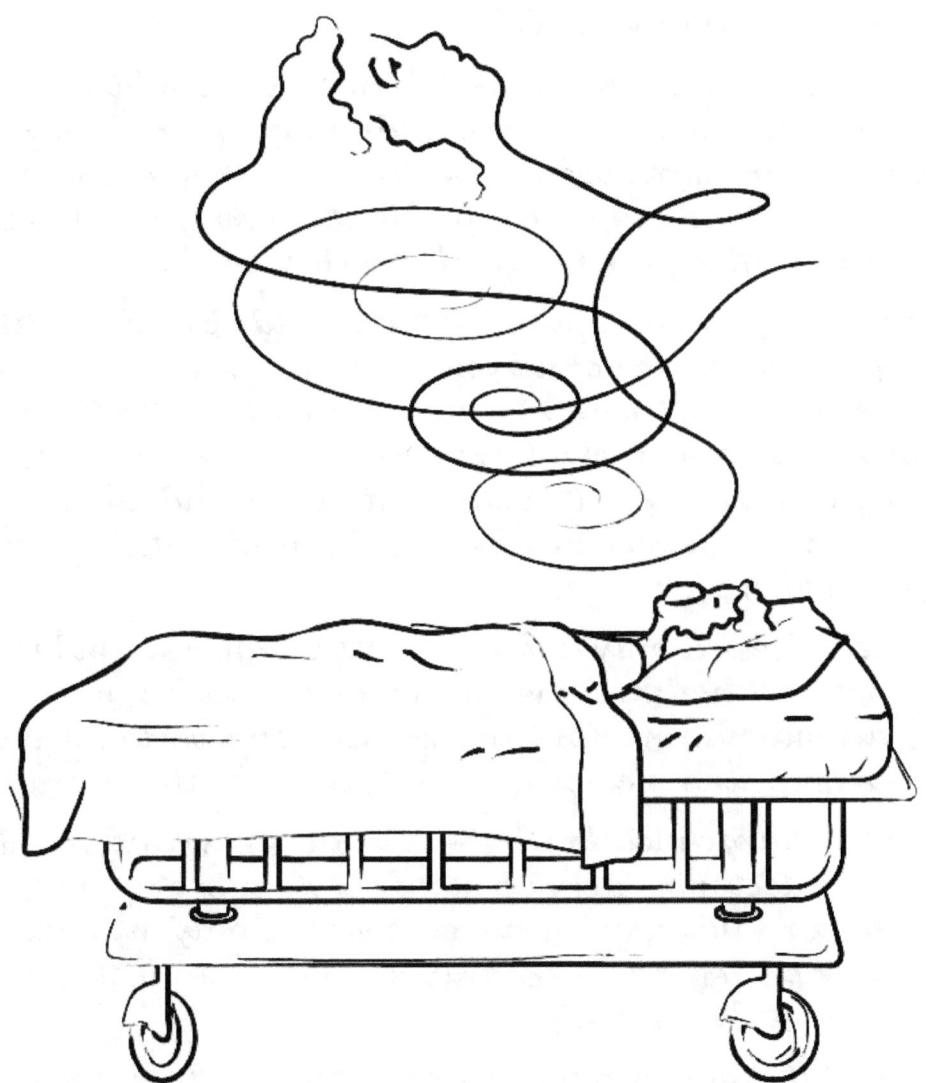

Memoirs

As I lie on a narrow cot, my throat is painful from swollen and angry tonsils. My skin is colorless, yet burning with fever, my hair dry and lifeless. My mother bends over me, murmuring incantations. She hovers, brushing her bare hand across my forehead and over my chest in soft caressing circles until my eyes close and my breathing slows.

When I awake, she feeds me steaming hot soups and teas with lemon and honey. Sometimes she adds a dollop of whiskey that tastes so vile I would rather be miserably sick then anywhere near it. Somehow I missed out on the proclivity of my Scottish heritage for appreciating the merits of good rye whiskey.

Soon I am sitting on a hospital stretcher - side by side - with another girl of same age of six years. We are wheeled into a large room. Several hands transfer me to another bed-like table. I know not where I am or why I am here. I only know I was brought here by my tight-lipped parents who handed me over to strangers. I hear the murmuring of soft sounds. Still no one tells me what I am here for.

I am chilled, dressed only in a thin, cotton gown. I am laid down, covered with a sheet over my body and with a mask of stinging aroma over my nose and mouth. The world spins in front of me, spinning me, spinning me, into another world...

I come to in a large metal crib. My throat is raw and painful from the tonsillectomy. I cry up blood, crying, crying out for my mother who does not come. I have no words, only my heart-wrenching cries. My cries turn into whimpers, and still my mother does not show herself.

Many weeks later, my throat is better, yet words do not rise easily. I have just come out of the tiny bathroom and into the large yellow kitchen. My mother stands over the stove, cooking our supper. She turns to me and says: "Bonnie, you are going to have to say good-bye to Mary. You are going to school now and you are too old to have an imaginary friend."

I hear my mother tell me that I must say goodbye to this friend whom I talk with often throughout the day. Yet, I do not understand; I am baffled in a swirl of confusion. I am lost in the churning for I am suddenly without an awareness of Mary.

I don't know where Mary is. In the years that follow, I occasionally imagine I hear her whisper. Especially when I am near the lake and in the woods. My favorite place is a small, moss-covered overhang, rich in pine and hemlock with an expansive view of the water far below. There I almost feel her Presence wrap around me, almost hear her murmuring in the velvet breezes, almost sense her in the moistness of the moss next to my skin. These times are like a brief kiss, a brush of the lips almost touching the skin. Most of the time I barely remember Mary.

My parents, brothers and sisters close the wood and glass paneled front door. It's a regular routine that we all go to Sunday school and worship at the steepled eighteenth century brick church. We sit on Shaker-styled wooden pews on the right side, tenth row down; Grandpa and Nana Johnson sit in the row behind. Grandpa McCrandles always stays at home. When I beg him to go with us, Grandpa McCrandles wryly replies, "If I went the church would fall in."

This year is different. I'm sick. Coughing and feeling tired all the time. I miss school for weeks on end, miss playing outside with my friends and miss real church. Instead, Sunday after Sunday, while the rest of my family heads off to church, I attend TV church. Wrapped in a worn hand-knitted afghan, I watch the altar calls and send a nickel in the mail to help support the crusades. One Sunday, when he invites us, including those of us watching at home, to commit our lives to God, I answer the call. I am ten and Mary is a faded memory. Yet maybe something in God's Presence within Billy Graham reminds me of the Presence of Mary. So I am drawn to this Presence, recognizing something that calls me. Yet, I don't trust God and I don't trust my mother and I don't trust any one in authority. But I don't know that yet.

Years later something nudges me. "What?" No answer, so I go back to doing whatever. Poke. "What?" Soon I am aware that, like a baby bird, I am being gently prodded out of the nest. I am being called to do God's work. "What work do you want me to do?" I ask. I hear: "Come. Commit to doing My Will. Then, you will know." "Are you kidding?" I respond, "Not on my life. You tell me first. What kind of work? Then I will tell you whether I will do it." SILENCE. Absolute Silence. I retort: "Okay be that way. I will figure out what to do without Your instructions." I tell myself: "Certainly I can figure how to do helpful things without God's help." I climb back in the center of the nest and cockily do <u>my</u> rendition of God's work. I am twenty years old and for the next twenty years the Great Spirit nudges and I don't budge. I will not commit to being thrown into a lion's den. I went to Sunday school and heard all those Bible stories about what happens to people who do God's bidding. No thanks to lion's dens, bellies of whales, arks crowded with animals, beheadings and worse. No!

I have cast God as the Persecutor and "poor me" as the Victim. I put on the mantle of Rescuer and do good works. I volunteer as Sunday school teacher, tutor children, help the poor, advocate for human rights and for peace, and nurse the sick. I attempt to practice what I think of as the basics of a spiritual way of being: loving others. It all sounds good and I pat myself on the back for being such a good person.

Having left Spirit by the wayside, my spiritual awareness is matter-of-fact. I live in the Newtonian world. Ideas, like walks on water, water turned into wine, and visitations by angelic beings, are all outside the "natural" mechanical laws so are not believable and of no consequence to me. "God will not break God's own laws" is my constant credo.

Then, what is this restless longing?

From Natural Mammal to Drama Dance

We leave behind the chapter on the natural mammal and enter the chapter on the Drama Dance Experience, including the process of how we became members in, what I sometimes call, the Three-Stepping Drama Dance Club. What follows is a story that bridges as well as contrasts the natural mammal of three-year-old Bonnie with the potential creation of the drama dance in ten-year-old Josephine.

A young slim girl of ten years crosses the street from her home -one story, four rooms, falling apart, seven children, alcoholic father, and cowering mother - to mine. At three years old, I am too young to know the vast stretches - No really, chasms - that separate her home from mine. Instead, I watch as she crosses, arms loosely by her side, head down, her light hidden deep in the background of her eyes. Slowly, she climbs the rough, paint-peeling wooden steps; shyly and with hesitation, she barely knocks on our back door. Somehow my mother hears her. "Can I baby-sit for you, Mrs. Johnson?"

My mother looks like Mrs. Cleaver of "Leave it to Beaver." Dressed in a worn housedress, covered with a simple, cotton apron, she is a stay-at-home mom who sees being a mother as a divine calling. She is as dedicated to this calling as the ancient priestesses were to Isis.

My mother's response still startles me almost sixty years later. To Josephine: "I don't really need anyone to care for my children."

(Even now, in my mind, I ask: "How can she say that?" She had four children, the youngest just a baby. I remember how many times as an adult, I felt pulled out of the turbulent sea of parenting by the reprieve of a babysitter!)

My mother continues to Josephine:: "If you want, you can play with Bonnie in the yard." So off Josephine and I go, small hand shelters tiny hand. We gather leaves into an unending mountain. We cover ourselves completely, burying ourselves into the crisp crunches, the warm layers, and the pungent smells. We revel in the sweet abandon of throwing leaves up into the air and over our bodies.

"Josephine, get over here right now!" The harsh call of Josephine's father turns her to trembling and me to running back to my mother.

When Josephine's father calls for Josephine, three-year-old Bonnie detected danger in the harsh voice of Josephine's father and in Josephine's trembling response and frightened eyes. Bonnie saw and felt danger and sought her protectors. She was scared and ran to a safe haven, full of adults who protected her from harm. She was able to notice she was scared and do something about it. She acted; she made something happen that benefited her.

But not so for Josephine who, when she recognized the danger in the harsh voice of her father, experienced helplessness. She was not able to make things happen to keep her safe. Her sense of being powerful diminished. She was on her way to learning the Drama Dance.

The Drama Dance

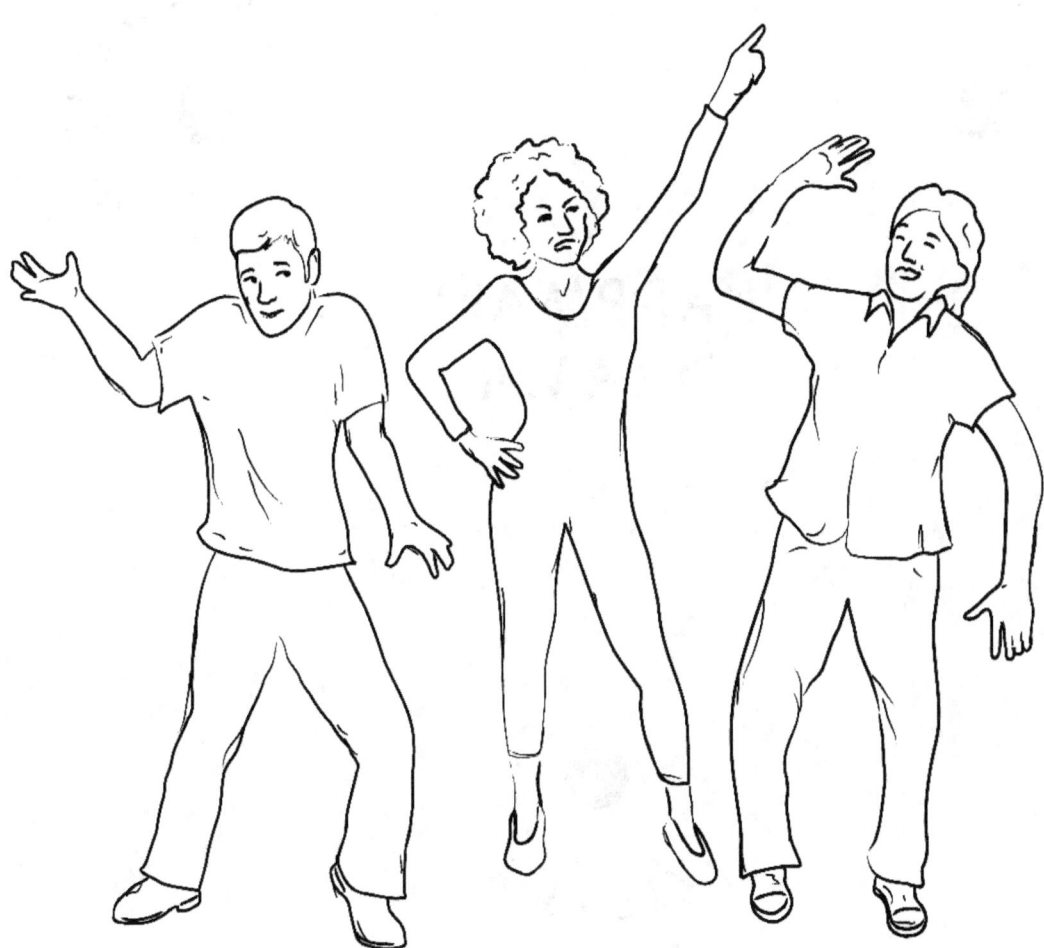

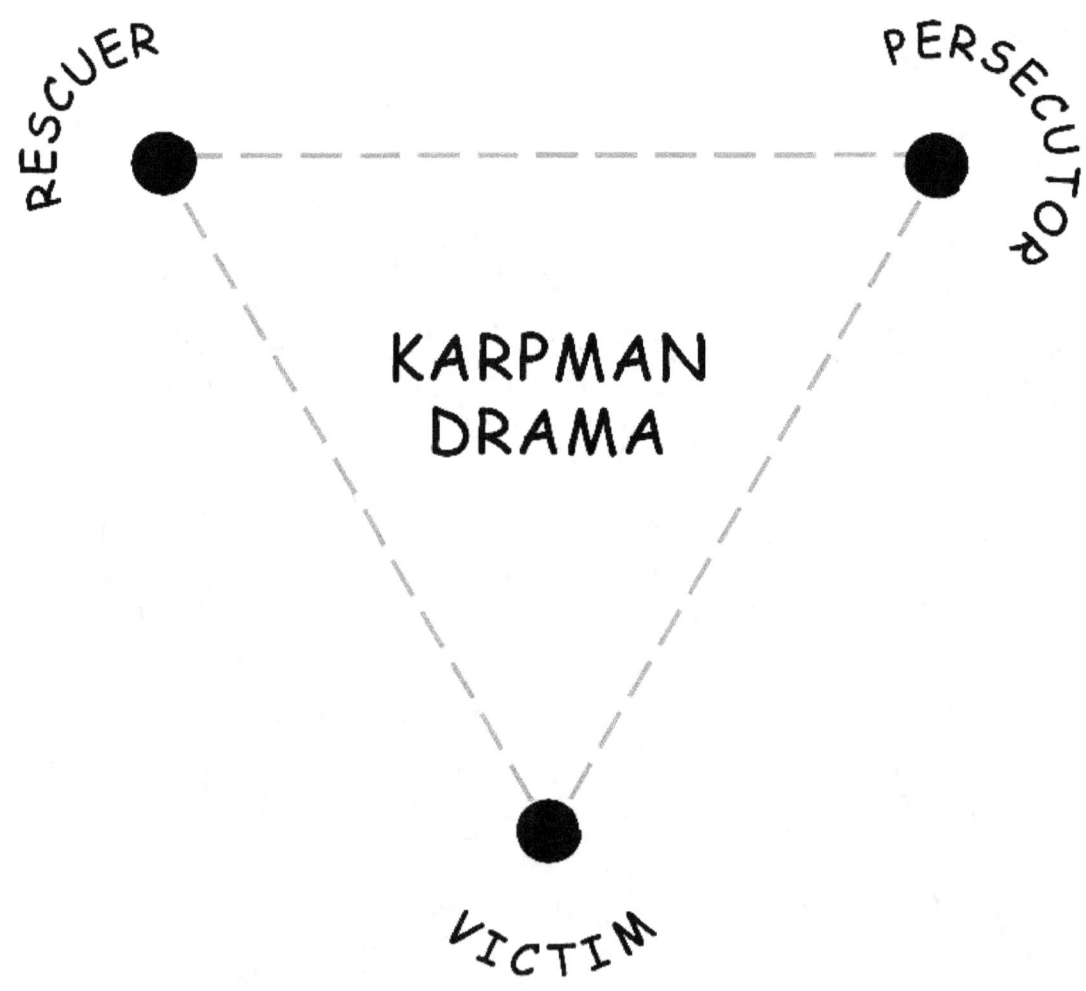

Prep Three:
Choosing a Drama Dance Experience

We have taken the first two preparation steps: the six-pointed star meditation and remembering a natural mammal experience. Now we continue the preparation with a Drama Dance experience. 1. Begin Prep Three by repeating the Six-Pointed Star Meditation. Recall that the six-pointed star is an energetic gateway through which transformational healing energies flow. By tracing it in our own energy systems we invite in those healing energies.

> **PREP THREE**
>
> ⚜ Repeat Six-Pointed Star Meditation.
>
> ⚜ Complete or Trace the drawing of the Victim-Rescuer-Persecutor Triangle.
>
> ⚜ Choose Drama Dance example in your life.
>
> ⚜ Experience an energetic healing technique. See pages 117-132.
>
> ⚜ Identify and write a word or sentence that describes you in each of the roles. Use the diagram: "Tips On Identifying The Three Roles" on page 59.
>
> ⚜ Use the VRP drawing to record this information.

2. Next complete the diagram of the Karpman Drama triangle on the next page. The completion of this diagram creates healing connections within our memories, bodies, and brains. For this triangle, use the color red, which energizes the vibration of red in your human energy system and aids in healing. Notice that both the Natural Mammal and the Karpman Drama triangles are drawn with the color red. Both are related to the root chakra and to feelings of trust, safety, security, survival and vitality.

3. Now **choose** a Drama Dance experience in your own life. You may find you need additional energetic support as you recall a drama dance experience. If so, **use the healing technique** *Shift in Consciousness Breathing* on page 127.

4. Then, i**dentify** and write a word or sentence that describes you in each of the roles. 5. Finally, **record** the above information on the VRP drawing.

Identification of the roles while in the Drama can be quite challenging as we are often in a trance state in which we are not aware of how we are behaving or what we are saying. This trance state harkens back to prior experiences of socializations and trauma. Many of those prior experiences are unresolved and still live within us. Therefore our ability to observe ourselves in the present moment in the Drama Dance is greatly decreased. To increase observation of the drama dance and to identify the three roles accurately, start by choosing a Drama scenario that occurred in the past, rather than in the present moment.

As the healing process of *Three Turns of the Kaleidoscope* is experienced, the ability to identify the roles while in a drama dance will increase. Recognizing the roles in a presently occurring Drama leads to being able to move instantly out of the Drama. Like a punctured balloon, the Drama runs out of energy to sustain itself. In its place, as the kaleidoscope turns, a whole way of being and relating comes alive.

Before identifying the roles in your Drama Dance, you may wish to read the sample of Prep Three and the in-depth descriptions of the Drama Dance that follow.

Sample Prep Three

Listen to Josephine as she shares her story of her Drama Dance:

> Yesterday was a beautiful day- sun bright, temperatures in the mid-seventies. I set out on my bike to the heated swimming pool where I have temporary privileges. A slight breeze brushes me clean. I am in the midst of clearing out sixty years of accumulated treasures from my parent's home and have given myself a day off. So I am in a "This is my day off; I am going to relax and enjoy myself" mode. When I get to the pool, it is full of children. Okay, they only take up the shallow end of the pool. The whole rest of the long deep end is empty and waiting. I get in, start in on my laid back float-swim-float-swim method and am enjoying the water.
>
> I have let the children's noises fade into the background. One of the mothers picks up her cell phone and makes a call. I overhear that her father is in the hospital and undergoing tests to check out a serious heart condition. I hear myself whine silently:

"Geez, wouldn't you just know. I have to pick a day in January to go swimming with a pool of children and stressed out adults with a sick father." Now I know this is classic inner victim stance. It is: "Poor me. Ain't my life awful? I am at the mercy of these people and all I wanted was a little peace and relaxation." I have just entered the Three-Stepping Drama Dance Studio. I start dancing like mad when I say (again to myself). "Oh, you poor thing. You have been working really hard for weeks and this happens." Then, in the most demeaning voice: "You are supposed to be such a nice person and here you are complaining when someone else is having real troubles. Shame on you! There must be something really wrong with you to think that!

To help magnify the roles of Victim, Rescuer, and Persecutor in Josephine's Drama Dance, let's diagram it. Compare this information with the "Tips On Identifying The Three Roles" on the next two pages.

Rescuer:

"Oh, you poor thing. You have been working really hard for weeks and this happens."

Persecutor:

"You are supposed to be such a nice person and here you are complaining when someone else is having real troubles. Shame on you!"

Victim:

"Geez, wouldn't you just know it! I have to pick a day in January to go swimming with a pool of children and stressed-out adults with a sick father!"

NOTES:

Diagram (Opposite Page)

TIPS ON IDENTIFYING THE THREE ROLES: VICTIM, RESCUER, PERSECUTOR

A person assumes and continues any and all of the roles (victim, rescuer, persecutor) when strong feelings and beliefs related to an experience combine and then result in the expressions/behaviors.

Tips on Identifying the Three Roles 59

Persecutor's Energetic Support

BELIEFS
Judges victim as flawed:
- in personality
- in character
- mentally
- emotionally
- spiritually

FEELINGS
Sees victim as:
- inadequate...useless
- stupid...worthless
- useless...scum
- helpless...hopeless

EXPRESSIONS
- Battering
- Criticism
- Accusations
- Sarcasm
- Temper tantrums
- Violence
- Cornering
- Blaming

Rescuer's Energetic Support

BELIEFS
Relates to victim as:
- incapable
- unable
- flawed

FEELINGS
- Guilt
- Pain/suffering
- Needed
- Helpless
- Hopeless

EXPRESSIONS
- Helpful
- Everyone's best friend
- Mr./Ms. Nice
- Martyr
- Makes excuses

Victim's Energetic Support

BELIEFS
- Incapable
- Unable
- Powerless
- Out-of-control
- Not responsible

FEELINGS
- Helplessness
- Hopelessness
- Blamed
- Shame
- Guilt

EXPRESSIONS
- Whining
- Complaining
- Pouting
- Pessimistic
- Cynical
- Depressed

Original diagram design by Nelson Villalobos and adapted by the author.
Source of information: "The Three Faces of Victim" by Lyn Forrest
www.lynneforrest.com/html/the_faces_of_victim.html

© 2008 Three Turns of a Kaleidoscope by Bonnie Johnson
Permission granted to duplicate for personal and educational purposes.

The Drama Dance: What is it?

Imagine that you hold in your hand a broken kaleidoscope. Inside, the three, tiny, triangular pieces of mirror are chipped, cloudy, and cracked. When you peer through the round hole to view the reflections, the image is garbled, confused, and out of focus.

The Drama Dance is a distortion—like looking through the broken kaleidoscope—of the natural mammal state. This distortion is brought about through unresolved experiences of trauma, socialization and domestication. By entering into the Drama, we unconsciously and unsuccessfully attempt to heal old wounds and traumas.[35] Here on the Drama Dance floor, we go into defensive, protective circles of feeling victimized and hopeless. Yet we hope this time to reclaim our powerful, capable and playful selves. Instead, we look through cracked and blurred mirrors and experience again and again ourselves as powerless, helpless and full of shame.

The Drama Dance, in Stephen Karpman's model, is portrayed as an interactive game. One-to-three people can "play" at one time and each "Player" assumes three roles—Victim, Rescuer and Persecutor. In addition, the roles switch quickly. For example, one minute I may be playing the Victim; in the next second I switch to the Persecutor role, which tumbles another or me into the Victim role. In a flash, I find myself Rescuing the Persecutor who is now the Victim. All three roles are a playing out of different portrayals of an internalized Victim.

> **KARPMAN DRAMA TRIANGLE**
> Victim-Rescuer-Persecutor
>
> - High Drama
> - An interactive Game
> - One to three Players
> - Players assume three roles
> - Roles shift and change
> - Misery and shame flourish
> - No one wins; everyone loses
> - A psychological & social model

The three roles can also be described in terms of feelings, beliefs and actions that power the performances. When playing the Victim, people feel helpless, believe they are powerless and behave by whining, pouting, or complaining,

---
[35] Peter Levine

using some variation of "Poor me!" The feelings and the beliefs feed the behaviors of each role. For example, when playing the victim role, the feeling of helplessness and the belief of "I am not capable" energize the behaviors of "complaining and whining."

Full of pain and suffering for others, the Rescuer perceives others as not capable of meeting their own needs. The Rescuer works hard to take care of the Victim. In playing the Drama game, the Rescuer is the favorite role, especially among helping professionals. In this role, a person receives much praise for being so good, for being such a Nice Person.

In playing the role of the Persecutor, we are disdainful toward the Victim; we see the Victim as useless and worthless. We believe that the Victim's problems are all due to their being flawed in some way. Blaming and accusing are standard behaviors of the Persecutor.

The Persecutor is perceived as the worst role in this game. Everyone may want to be the Rescuer but hardly any one readily admits to being the Persecutor. So much so that people frequently and vehemently <u>deny</u> playing this role. People say: "Sure, I play the Victim and I know I am always Rescuing people who really don't need my help, but I never act like a persecutor. I am way too nice." Deny we may, but it doesn't change the truth: according to Karpman, once we jump onto the Drama Dance floor, all three roles are required. A Rescuer begets a Victim begets a Persecutor begets a Victim begets a Rescuer….

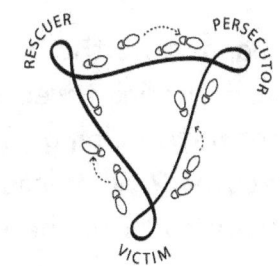

Like a three-stepping drama dance, this role switching can be likened to a fast moving whirl of changing dance steps and changing positions, with much bumping into others and stepping on each others' toes! The Victim cries "Poor me!" The Rescuer grovels: "I'm sorry. Poor you!" while putting ice on everyone's toes. The Persecutor, while still stepping on the Victim's toes, yells: "You clumsy oaf. Why don't you learn to dance?"

In naming the roles, Karpman gave us a way to bring this constellation of feelings, thoughts and behaviors to our awareness. When we name something, we provide a way for our unconscious mind to bring the hidden to the surface and to our awake consciousness. Naming helps us sift through the many, and isolate something that requires a more in-depth examination. Additional descriptors, such as Sufferer or Wounded or Blamed, name and therefore add additional light to the Victim role. Champion or Savior or Excuser reveals the Rescuer; Batterer or Tormentor or Blamer exposes the Persecutor.

Victim	Rescuer	Persecutor
Blamed	Excuser	Blamer
Sufferer	Savior	Tormentor
Wounded	Champion	Batterer

Using more names for the Drama encourages a more complete understanding of the many facets of the roles we assume and the variety of steps we (and our partners) dance.

Process of Becoming a Member of Three-Stepping Drama Dance Club

> *One of the pitfalls of childhood is that one doesn't have to understand something to feel it. By the time the mind is able to comprehend what has happened, the wounds of the heart are already too deep.*[36]   *Carlos Ruiz Zafon*

What happens to the beautiful, free-spirited child in all of us that generates a self-perpetuating three-stepping dancer of powerlessness (Sufferer/Victim), inappropriate-helping (Savior/ Rescuer) and devastating criticism (Tormentor /Persecutor)? What causes the natural mammal to undergo the distortion that gives birth to the Victim within?

In the ideal world, loving and supportive caregivers safeguard children until they are old enough and knowledgeable enough to protect themselves. Alas, this is not the ideal but the real world in which the natural mammal, unprotected by caregivers, encounters real hurt, real loss and real danger.

---

[36] Carlos Ruiz Zafon p.35

Even worse, sometimes the natural mammal endures danger and harm caused and aggravated by the caregivers.

Graud gives us a clue: "From infancy on, each of us undergoes a process of systematic indoctrination that turns us into socialized personalities… This process produces mixed results. We become proficient and complex personalities in a socialized world, but our indigenous self (natural mammal) is mostly lost to us and our access to its extraordinary intuitive and physical gifts, its dynamic vitality, and its innate connection to nature are severely diminished." [37]

The experience of being trained, programmed, conditioned, domesticated, and socialized distorts the natural process of learning and growing. It alters the way young children grow and learn through play. It short-circuits the way that they come to know their own abilities to make things happen. The adult, as teacher, provides this conditioning in the same way that many animals are domesticated: through punishments and rewards. Children often are punished for mistakes and rewarded for successes. Through this punishment/reward system, children become seekers of approval that brings rewards and avoiders of disparagement that spawns punishment. Therefore, children often begin to believe that they are good when rewarded and bad when punished.

To this distorted system of domestication, we add the unfair practices of already hurting adults who are in charge of domestication. These adults are inconsistent in their interactions with children. Many times, children feel they are punished for something they did not deserve. This unfairness creates stress and fear of the uncertainty and randomness of the domestication process.

Children grow afraid of learning, afraid of not getting rewards, and afraid of being punished. Because they cannot understand the complexities of this programming, they may blame themselves for their failure to get the rewards or for being punished. They often have distorted thoughts and beliefs: "I deserve to be punished." "Something is wrong with me." "The adults are right, so I am wrong." To compound these distorted thoughts, the adults pronounce judgments: "You are bad." And "What's wrong with you?" [38]

---

[37] Connie Graud p.20 & 24

[38] Adapted from a handout developed by Nelson Villalobos for the first "Healing the Inner Victim" workshop. Sources: The Four Agreements and The Mastery of Love by Don Miguel Ruiz

Dr. Charles Whitfield concurs: "With the help of parents, other authority figures, and institutions (such as education, organized religion, politics, the media, and even psychotherapy), most of us learn to stifle or deny our Child Within."[39] Slowly, children learn the art of pleasing their domesticators as is depicted in the following story:

> *Splashes and streaks of hot pink interlace with pure azure. The sun is just sinking below the ocean when I encounter the two brothers. They have unearthed a deep pit in the snowy sand. One brother, tired of his creative efforts, has returned to his parents. The five-year-old gazes at the pit with a glint in his eye. His whole attention is on the hole and the rising urges within him. In a flash, he throws up his arms and legs and hurls himself into the depression. In mid-flight, joy ripples through him. Landing, his abandon brings self-powered bliss. I laugh with the free joy so contagious in the presence of unbridled ecstasy. His slightly older brother, who has witnessed this spontaneous combustion of harmonic delights, runs over in hopes of capturing some. As he approaches, his eyes glance back and forth between the pit and me. He studies the pit for just the right way to jump and he studies me for the signal that he's doing it right. I am still in enjoyment from witnessing his younger brother as the older boy thoughtfully and with just a hint of rigidity, jumps into the pit. Before he has even landed, he looks to me for approval. I smile but he knows and I know that his jump is all out of kilter - missing the free-fall of natural play. The younger brother is living enjoyment; the older works to obtain the sufficient chits necessary to buy it. Yes, even children know that joy cannot be bought.*

---

39 Charles L. Whitfield p.9

With the unfair system of punishment and rewards (which usually results in pain, shame, guilt, and fear), the stage is set for the distorted version of the natural mammal triangle, as shown in the diagram[40] below.

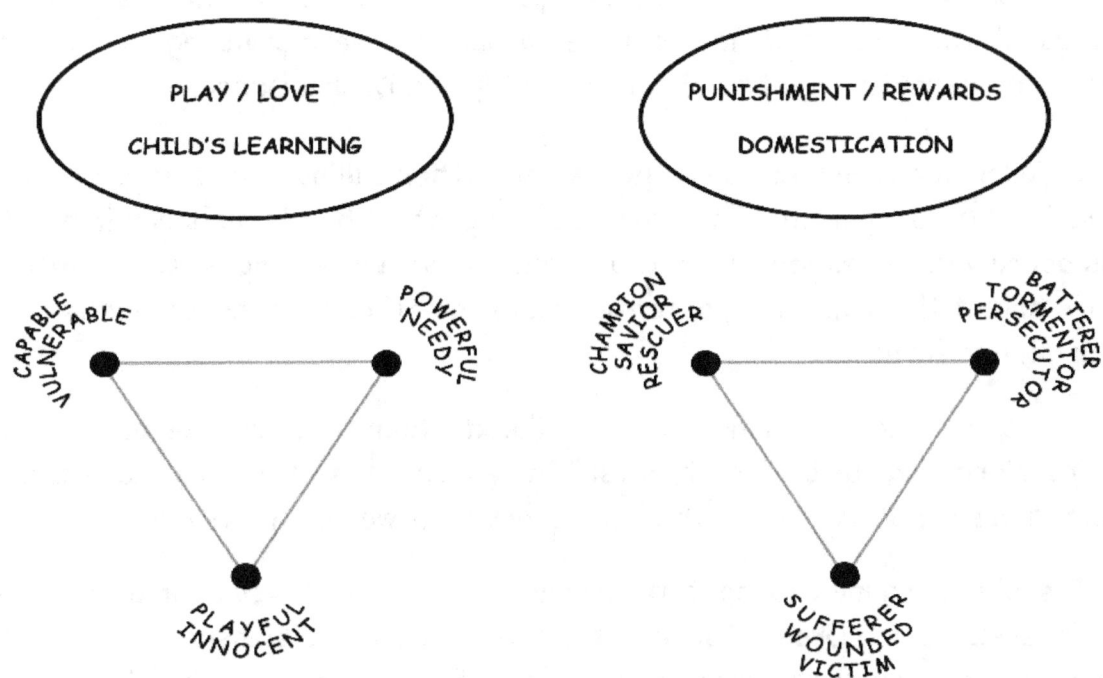

To these "normal" growing up experiences, add a long list of traumas people experience in being alive in the modern world: injuries, illnesses, surgeries, deaths and other losses, neglect, abuse—physical, emotional, mental, verbal, religious, institutional—and exposure to violence (real and imaginary).

By the time I am six years old, I have experienced years of being physically ill (probably from wheat and dairy consumption: a subtle trauma in itself), two surgical adenoidectomies and one tonsillectomy, the one year absence of my father during WW II, the loss of my mother's attention to care for my younger brother who is sicker than I am and the departure of my spirit guide, Mary. This does not include the "normal" traumas of going to school where my first-grade teacher put bags over the heads of children who disobeyed her, being hit on the head by a big ten year old trying to get back at my older brother, nor the frequent screaming of my mother as she released stress related to getting a pack of kids to do her bidding. Yet, all in all, I had a

---

40 Adapted from a handout developed by Nelson Villalobos for the first "Healing the Inner Victim" workshop. Sources: The Four Agreements and The Mastery of Love by Don Miguel Ruiz

happy childhood, loved by and living with two parents, two grandparents, in a large home with plenty of food, clothes, toys, friends, and immersed in a loving church community.

But all those traumas set in motion a propensity to dance the three-step. Besides, all the adults and older children around me were swinging and twirling to the out-of-rhythm beat of the Three-Stepping Drama Dance.

When Josephine trembles as she hears her father calling, she is experiencing a relationship to a parent who is supposed to protect her from harm; instead he is perceived and experienced as a threat to her well-being, seen as both unsafe and at the same time, potentially and sometimes protector. He is, after all, her father.

Josephine and I are not alone in our childhood experiences of trauma. Naparstek reminds us of the effects: "The essential insult of trauma is the helplessness it generates and the inadequacy that we feel in its grip."[41]

For Josephine and me and most of humanity, the stage was set for us to learn the Three-Stepping Drama Dance. It is that sense of helplessness, powerlessness, hopelessness that engenders the internalization of the victim. Remember, the natural mammal, when it encounters danger, either seeks protection from the adult caregivers or protects itself with learned skills. When harm threatens and we have neither the skills nor the ability to defend or protect ourselves, we experience being trapped with no way to be safe. Helplessness and hopelessness ensue.

The dogs on the beach, described earlier, often were trapped inside, no way to express their natural mammal drive to run, leap and twirl. They had learned to be quiet (that is good) in the house in hopes of a reward. Let loose on the beach, they quickly knew what to do. The natural mammal chooses play!

After attending a long and deadening event, Harvey describes a situation similar to the dogs: "On the walk home, I tried to revive myself (re-alive myself) by whooping and hollering, jumping up and down and waving my arms... It felt like my soul/spirit had been compressed, and I needed to expand it back out to its normal size."[42]

---

[41] Belleruth Naparstek p. 39

[42] Harvey Baker Personal communication January 2007

In the day-to-day life experiences, we are compressed by our environment and then let loose to expand back out to normal size. This happens countless times in our childhood and adult life. Yet, trauma—little and big—is cumulative and embodied. Some little thing – a movement, aroma, voice tone, color, song, building, chair, texture, or touch, hurtles us back into a time where we experienced profound helplessness. There we may become suffering victims and act out of that modus operandi. Because we have been taught (in word, model and invitation) to dance the three-step whenever we experience helplessness, we respond to this helpless memory by dancing out of rhythm. We either dance with our inner partners or we easily find 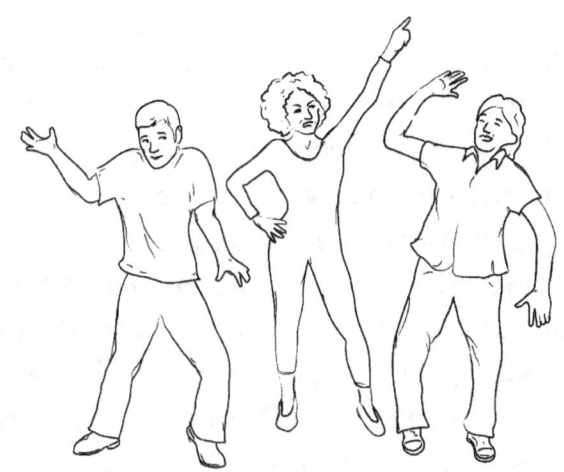 outer partners who personify the "blink-of-an eye" switching from victim to champion to batterer. We know the steps and our partners well, and we know that being out of rhythm and stepping on toes are essential requisites for this dance. We dance intensely, yet nothing changes.

The Attraction and Perpetuation of the Drama Dance, or Paying Dance Club Dues

the soul …never stops calling us back to our birthright integrity [43]
Parker Palmer

When we are living the drama dance, the experience can be likened to being pulled down deeper and deeper into the miry swamp of our distorted views. When we keep our attention on the drama, trying to solve the drama, we keep ourselves in the swirl and stomp of going nowhere but into deepening misery. We persevere in a process that neurologist Robert Scaer calls "kindling." He defines kindling as "…**internal** *(bold added)* cues of the trauma (that) become part of the source for arousal related to a specific trauma event." [44] This kindling (as in twigs that catch fire and burn up quickly) occurs not because of a current external traumatic or dangerous event. Instead, it is a quantum quick response to inner chemical changes that are lived as an inner scenario plays out over and over.

Connie Graud puts it this way: "If a jaguar crosses your path, fear gives you energy to take appropriate action, like running away. But once you have taken action and you're out of danger, it doesn't help to keep re-imagining the event, or to imagine the jaguar actually eating you. To keep fear alive in your mind and your body is…a loss of soul and with it, a loss of energy." [45] Frank MacEowen in *The Mist-Filled Path* observes "…the individual suffering from soul loss does not have full access to their soul's energy, vitality, memory, or inspiration for living." [46]

Naperstek devotes a whole chapter—"Frannie's Story: A Humbled Therapist's Education"—to the kindling effects of telling our traumatic story one more time. She relates:

> Not only did the intensity of these episodes (flashbacks or re-experiences of the original trauma) fail to dissipate with their retelling; if anything, they seemed to be getting worse…My experience

---

43 Parker J. Palmer p.58
44 Robert Scaer p. 62
45 Connie Graud p.18-20
46 Frank MacEowen p. 25

and training... had ...led me to believe that as people shared the horror of their experience with a trusted, empathic, but neutral listener, its intensity would evaporate... This did not happen with Frannie.[47]

When we tell our story immersed in the drama dance, we re-kindle and re-live ourselves as Victim. Therefore we add fire to the drama.

Several years ago, I was part of a group in which one person triggered the drama dance in me. Each time I returned home from being with this group, I would share my story including my frustrations with my husband Rich. As the months passed and I continued to tell this same story of woe, swirling and twirling myself dizzy, Rich's interest in listening and helping exhausted itself. One day, after several minutes of listening to the "same old story," he announced clearly and emphatically that he would no longer listen. In that second, where multiple worlds were suspended, I felt angry that he could be so callous AND I became aware that continued talking about this situation was making it worse, not better. I could see that I had cast us all in the inner victim roles that only created misery and led us away from the peace and love and joy we seek.

When we tell our story from the perspective of self-prescribed Victim-Rescuer-Persecutor, we wrap ourselves in vines that bind, cut, tangle and pull us deeper into the swamp of misery.

This is not to discard or diminish the therapeutic effects of being listened to as we speak aloud our story. This is to alert us to the potential danger in activating the kindling: the arousal that is once again experienced in body and spirit, just as in the original trauma. In addition, there comes a time, when the story has been told and we have reaped the healing that comes from telling. When that time comes and we continue to tell the story, we energize the effects of the original traumas; we keep ourselves in the drama and we are often clueless as to why things are not improving in our life. This is the exact opposite of what we are reaching for. So instead of the carousel's golden ring, we grasp a rusty barbed wire that cuts and wounds again!

---

47 Belleruth Naparstek p.19

Complete or Modify Prep Three

After reading this chapter on the Drama Dance you may need or want to return to pages 54-55 and reread the directions for third preparatory step. If you have not completed Prep Three, do so now. If you have, you may wish to make some changes.

Review and Summary of Prep Three

Three Turns of a Kaleidoscope: Healing The Victim Within

PREP ONE
  Do the Six-Pointed Star Meditation.
PREP TWO
  Identify one Natural Mammal Triangle experience in your own life.

PREP THREE
1. Repeat the Six-Pointed Star Meditation.
2. Complete the drawing of the Victim-Rescuer-Persecutor Triangle.
3. Choose one Drama Dance experience in your own life.
4. Experience an energetic healing technique.
5. Identify and write a sentence that describes you in each of the roles.
6. Record this information on the VRP drawing.

Move to Part IV: Initiation and the first, second and third turns of the kaleidoscope.

Part IV: INITIATION

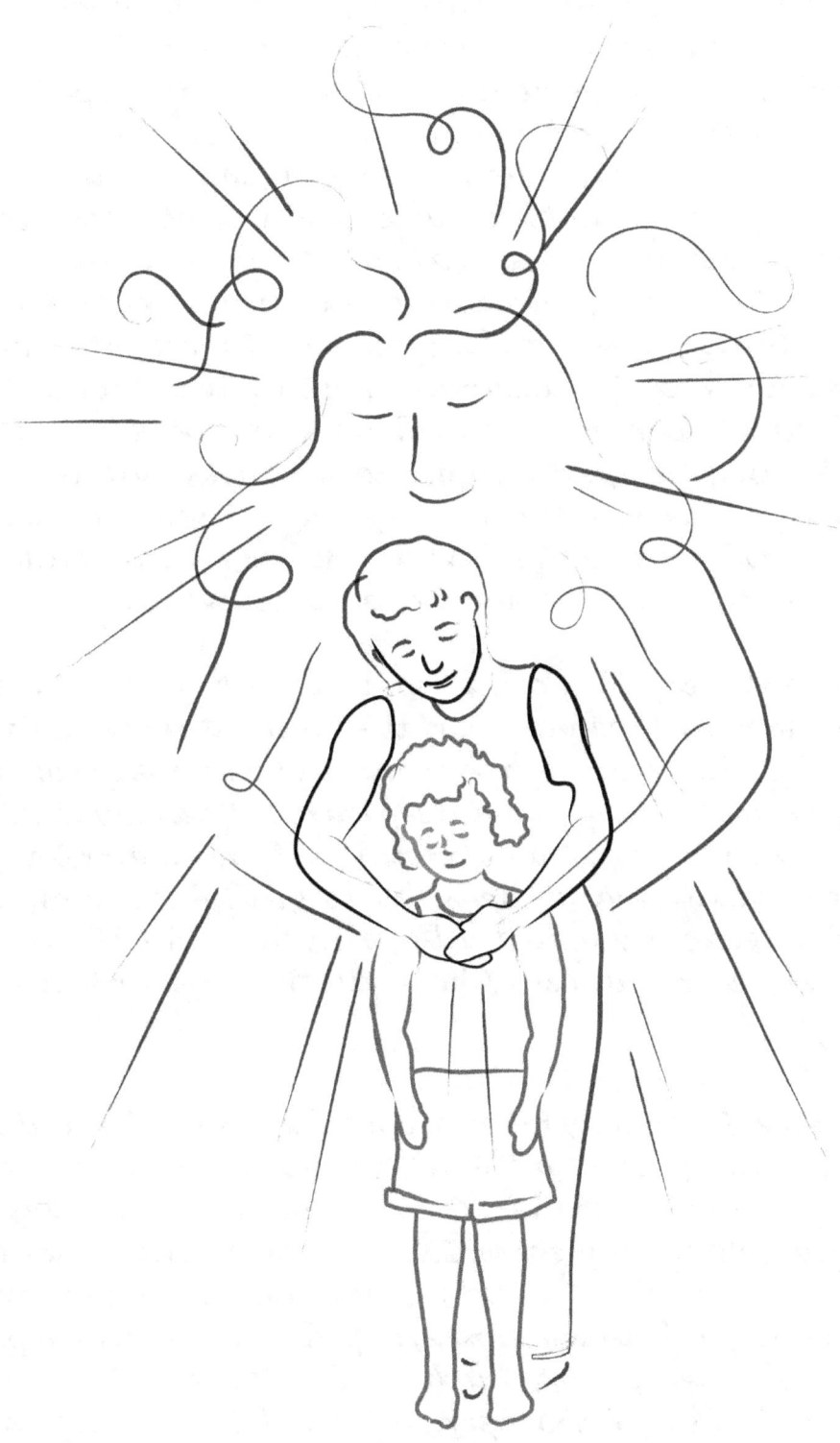

Memoirs 1980's Nashville, Tennessee

Something begins to change. The longing gets stronger. Urgings pull at me to explore and to come to a deeper understanding of my own beliefs and reconcile them with my spiritual path and living. I decide to go on a spiritual journey for one year. In order to do this, I must juggle my life as a single mother of three children, my job as a full time nurse, and my volunteer work at the church. Something has to give, so I take a one-year "sabbatical" from church work, one year that turns into many years. Deeply and passionately, I journey. I meet with an older, wiser woman who easily helps me explore my unorthodox beliefs and un-beliefs. I converse with a friend who serves as my spiritual director/advisor. She places in my hands books that describe other worlds: writings by Ruth Montgomery, Edgar Cayce and Raymond Moody. I am sure she has lost her mind. Gently, she encourages me to read them so we can discuss the ideas.

As I step into these other worlds - some describe this as standing on the threshold between the worlds - I am entranced. The Newtonian world can no longer contain me. I have crossed into spiritual realms that quench a deep thirst. When my spiritual director and I meet again, my mouth and mind go non-stop with all the new teachings and ideas. We toss insights and meanings back and forth across a spiritual net. In the midst of our discussions, she announces: "I have just the book for you. I will send it to you."

Back at home, I promptly forgot about the book. The nudges start again and I recognize that "God" is calling me. For some mysterious reason, I respond, "Okay. I am willing. Whatever You direct, I will follow." Somehow, I speak these words without hesitation or fear. This "yes" sets something new in motion. Within forty-eight hours a book wrapped in plain brown paper arrives. It is "Therapeutic Touch: How to Use your Hands to Help and to Heal" by Dolores Krieger. As I read, I know instantly that this is my life calling. I now know that all those pokes and proddings over the past twenty years were urging me toward hands-on healing!

Yet another surprise awaits me. A child development colleague beseeches me, "I need your help. A three-year old in one of the preschool classes has an imaginary friend. The parents are worried about her because she talks and plays with this 'friend'. What do you know about imaginary friends?" I tell her what I know, and then add, "Be respectful and gentle and honor the child's relationship to the imaginary friend. This is really important to do because the imaginary friend is an essential part of the child." As I hear myself speaking these words, I am stunned.

As my professional self finishes the call and hangs up, my six-year-old self appears before me, bereft of her essential self. We look at each other. Somehow, I know what to do. I reach out to my six-year-old self and bring her close to me. I turn slightly and speak these words of invitation: "Mary, wherever you are, please come back. I am sorry I ever sent you away. Please return." Instantly, I am aware of the Presence of Mary. My six-year-old self and I breathe a deep sigh of rightness. "Where have you been? Why did you leave me?" cries my six-year-old self. Mary answers: "I have been right here with you. I never left you. It is you who turned from me. I am with you always."

Every day, I am aware of Mary's Presence and Her Guidance. As the years unfold I continue my study and practice of hands-on energetic healing. The wound that began long ago when I said goodbye to Mary starts to heal. I begin to trust "God/dess," I begin to trust myself and to recognize my own inner authority. The old ways die; new ways emerge; life flourishes. In the midst of this, She begins to teach me new healing ways: ways that are needed for this time; ways that bring in the healing energy that will mend the male/female divisions; ways that assist humanity to claim its true spiritual nature; ways that return us all to the Great Cosmic Mother; ways that transform and transcend our limitations, our internal prisons, our self-imposed rules; ways that open up the heavens and usher us in.

One day the bottom drops out of my life. My eighteen-year-old son is sent to prison. My father has a stroke; my sister dies of cancer within six months of diagnosis; my mother has a heart attack, a stroke, and dies; my relationship with my husband totters and flounders. I rail against this God that I never did trust. I tell Him that this whole human life stuff is a crummy system and I could come up with a better plan. I am so angry with God. Someone tells me "Well, at least you are still speaking." "Oh! I am definitely speaking! I have truly told God what I think. I am crying, yelling, ranting and raving. I come face to face with all that pain inside of me - pain at being betrayed and abandoned - pain of being a Victim - a "poor me" look what life has done to me and look what the Great Persecutor has done and not done. Ugly old "pus" comes pouring out of me.

My son gets out of prison and we all go to family therapy. The therapist asks: "Who makes the decisions in the family?" Everyone turns to and points at me. I am totally baffled. "Me? I never get my way. I do what everyone else wants. You all never do what I want." They all look at me as if I am crazy. They say in unison: "If you don't want something to happen, it won't. You get the final say so." I whisper: "Oh, that's true." I am humbled by this power. I have seen myself as the Victim for so long, I forgot I carried a big power club in my hands, which I wield amazingly well. Once upon a time I would have dropped the club like a hot potato. I would have been too scared to admit I could exercise that much personal power. I would have been frozen with horror at the very thought. This time I feel my chest expand, my head stretch upward, my mouth turn into a surprised and happy grin. I hold the club, testing its weight, grateful for its substance and fortitude. Slowly, I put it down, confident it will be there when I need it. I turn to my family and say with conviction, "Yes, that's true."

The pus finally is all out and I can see a clean wound. I attend the wound with a tenderness usually reserved for others. I begin to stop looking for others to take care of my wounds - but I have just started on this part of my journey: healing the Victim within.

Three Turns: Three Healing Triangles

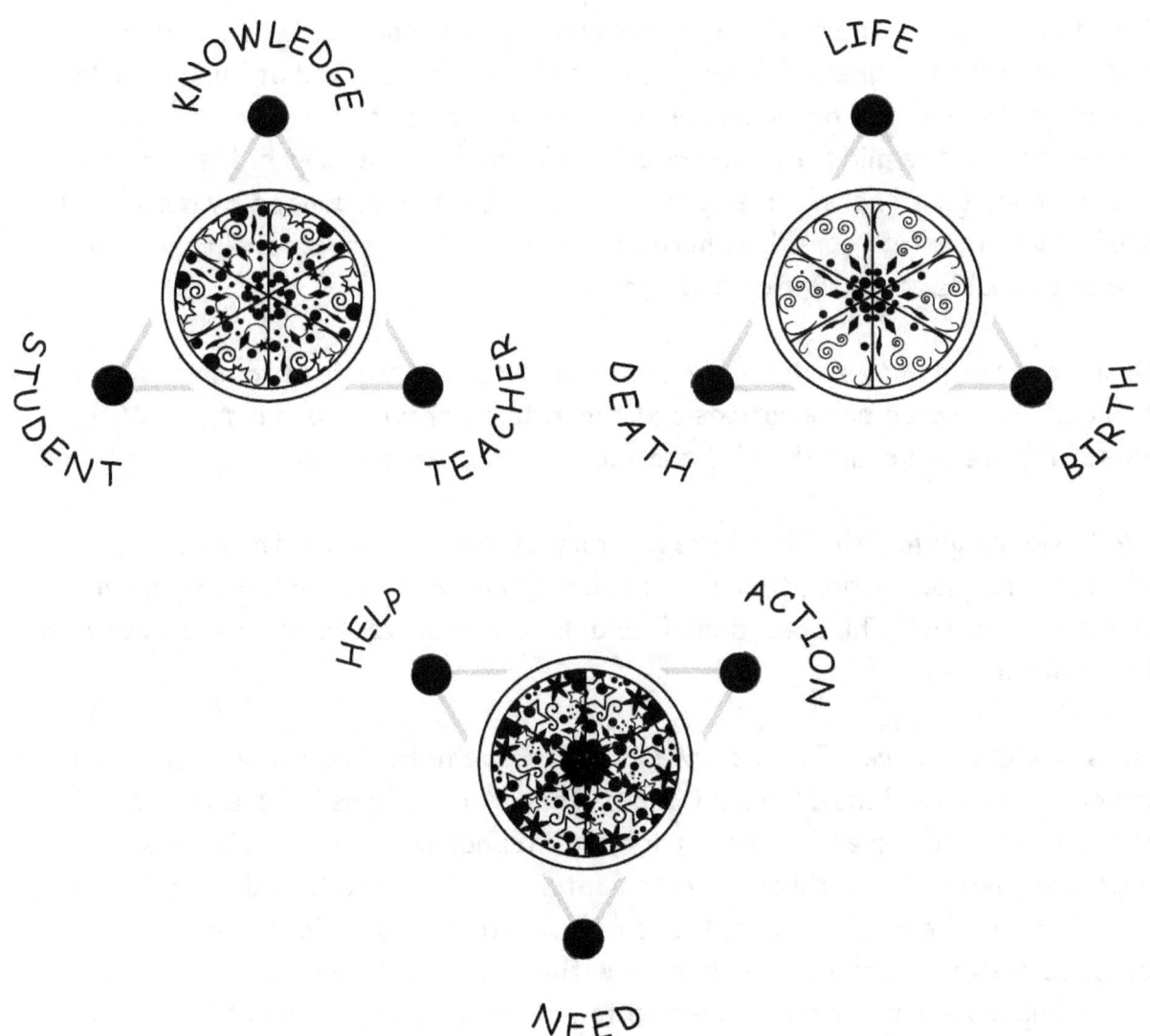

Stop Paying Your Dues: The Way Out – Resigning Membership in the Drama Dance Club

Something within us can transform suffering into wisdom.
Rachel Naomi Remen

The Drama Dance serves as a launching pad, not an end point. Graud writes "...shamans believe the soul sometimes chooses pain and disillusionment in order to grow into greater wholeness. An old life is sloughed off like a snake shedding its skin, and a new and greater life is revealed. But the soul must choose this in the midst of the ordeal." Herein lies the DD's hidden treasure: the diamond gem, transformed after years of being surrounded by dark thick stuff. When we find ourselves mired in the ordeal of drama dancing, we can (we are capable of this!) stop and choose.

Graud goes on to say that a shift in consciousness is required to make such a choice.[48] The three preparations and three turns provide such a shift. With this shift, we can claim the gift that our soul has brought us.

We have completed the three preparatory steps beginning with the Six-Pointed Star Meditation, then we recalled a time when our natural mammal was alive and well. Third we identified a drama dance experience from our own life experiences.

Let's now apply *Three Turns of the Kaleidoscope* to healing the victim within in yours and Josephine's Drama Dance. These three turns involve the use of three healing triangles (previous page). Metaphorically, these triangles represent each of the three mirrors contained within the kaleidoscope. With each turn of the kaleidoscope, these mirrors/triangles reflect new perspectives that can create changes within us. The kaleidoscopic approach to healing moves us from out-of-step to rhythmic dancing, from freezing to freeing, from compressed to expanded, from suffering to joy, from blaming to celebrating, and from repeating the old to creating and recreating new ways of living in this moment.

---

48 Graud and Childers p.167

First Turn

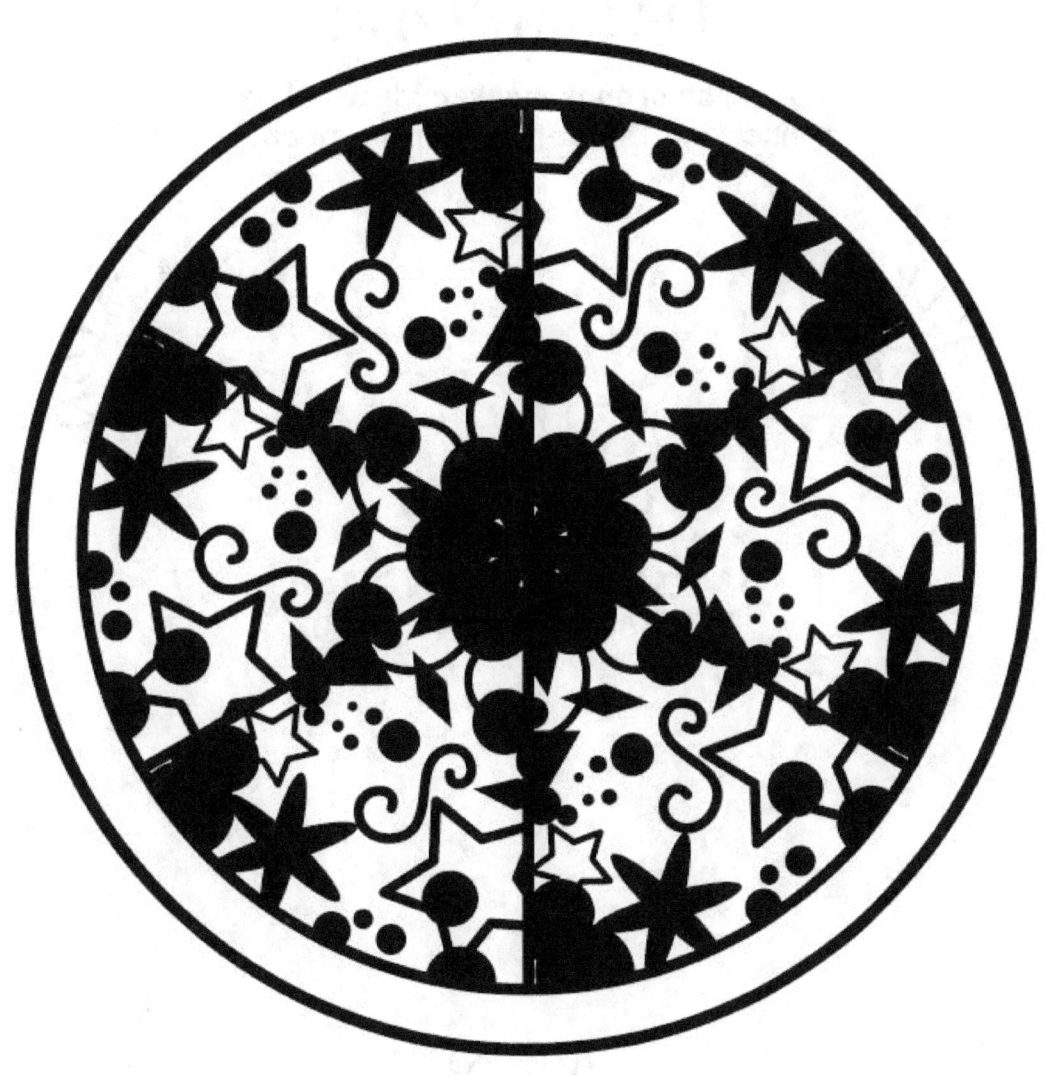

THE NEED-ACTION-HELP TRIANGLE

Using an orange marker, draw a line connecting the dots to form a triangle

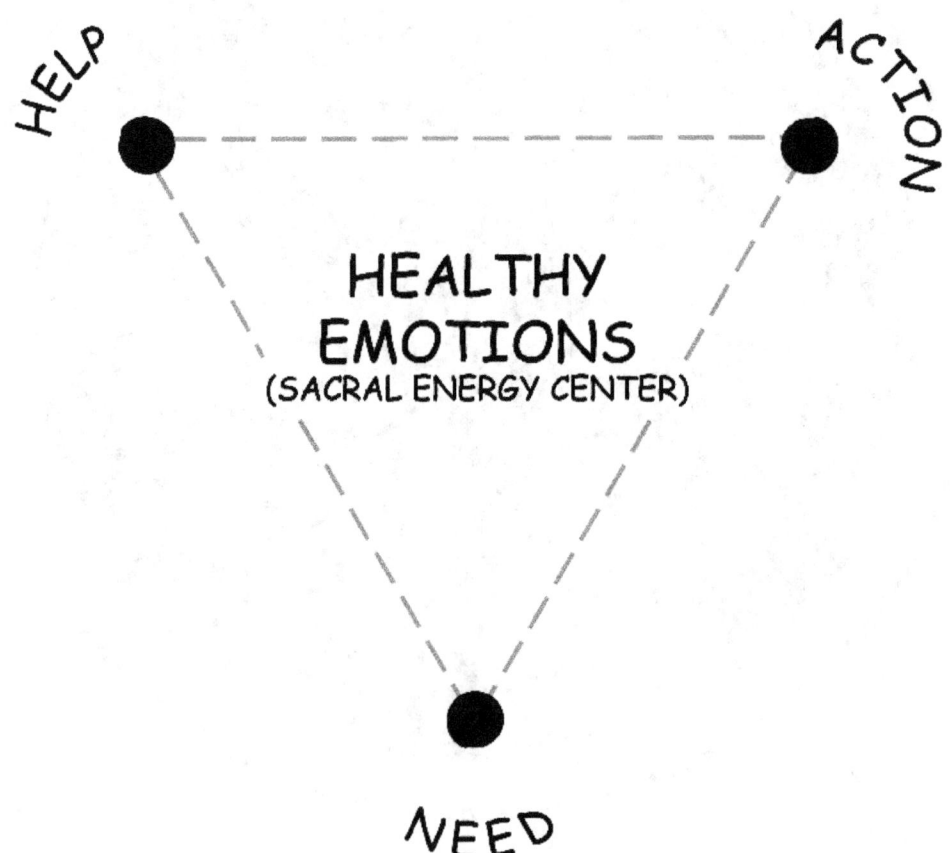

First Turn: Becoming Safe

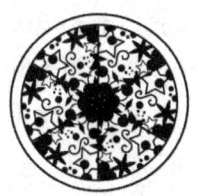

FIRST TURN

- Complete Need-Help-Action Triangle drawing.

- Repeat the Six-Pointed Star Meditation.

- Using your Drama Dance experience:

  Identify the Need. When we step onto the Drama Dance (DD) floor, what need are we trying to meet? The answer to the question has something to do with safety, survival, security, trust, and vitality. What is the need?

  Identify the Help. Examine what help is required to meet the identified need. Choose from three transformational tools: self-love, forgiveness or truth. What is the help?

  Identify the Action. Ask what action is needed to meet the identified need with help of the identified tool. Note: Answer with first thought and briefly.

- Choose a word or sentence that encapsulates your answers. Use the NHA drawing to record this information.

- Experience an energetic healing technique as needed.

Start the First Turn by
1. Completing the drawing of the Need-Help-Action triangle, which is the first healing triangle. Like the drama triangle, this triangle, is drawn with apex pointing downward. In the drama triangle, the downward point suggests distorted energies of being mired or stuck. However, in the Need-Help-Action triangle, the downward point conveys the healthy energies of stability and grounding.

Using the color orange helps to connect to the energetic vibrations of the second energy center and the healing qualities of balance and creativity. As the first turn of the kaleidoscope, the Need-Help-Action Triangle forms the ground of experiences for shifting from unconscious defensive existence to self-aware, freely choosing living.

To facilitate this shift, put down that broken kaleidoscope you have in your hand.

Now, imagine that you are looking through a new, beautifully made kaleidoscope with three mirrors that are made of the best reflective material and are clear and intact. As you look through the viewer, turning the dial, a pattern appears that is clear, vibrant and humbling in its aesthetic beauty.

This pattern is a reflection of the first of the three mirrors inside the kaleidoscope. This first triangular-shaped mirror, the Need-Help-Action Triangle, provides clear and easily followed guidelines for right choices. It helps us move out of our unconscious defense patterns of retreating into underground hideouts; walling ourselves in and everyone else out; attacking with scathing words; or dismissing or minimizing hurtful behaviors. This healing reflection helps us to discover what the distorted drama and dancing is all about. From this point of discovery, we can be awake to our basic needs and actually choose care for those needs with respectful attention.

The Need-Help-Action Triangle through the Eyes of the Human Energy System

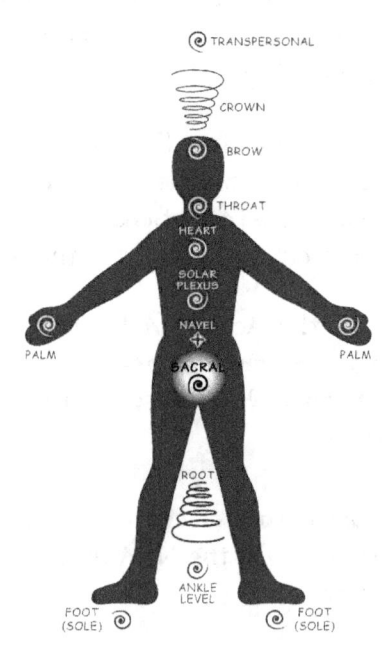

This healing triangle is associated with the energy of the second chakra: the sacral energy center, located at the level of the sacrum (the flat bone at the base of the spine, just above the tailbone) and the lower abdomen (below the navel). This chakra processes energetic information that is related to ordinary objects, actions and emotions, and to balancing opposites in the same space.

Ordinary, as used here, can best be described as related to a certain vibrational range that we recognize as things: our bodies, pencils, chairs, tables, stones, or dirt as well as certain emotions. Clairvoyants see this vibrational

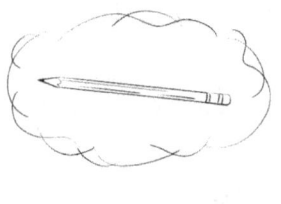

range usually in the red-orange-yellow spectrum and our ears recognize it as the musical tones C, D or E. A pencil in material form vibrates at a low (slow) frequency. The **idea** of a pencil vibrates at a different (faster) frequency than the pencil in material form. Ordinary emotions vibrate at slower (not as slow as material objects) frequencies than extraordinary emotions. Ordinary emotions (sad, glad) are grounding and help keep our attention earth bound; extraordinary emotions (empathy, bliss) are experienced as uplifting, transforming and transcendent.

Both Ordinary **and** Extraordinary emotions are necessary for our full experience as humans. However, the ordinary emotions are the province of the sacral energy center.

The balancing of opposites, by way of the healthy sacral chakra energies, occurs without either quality (such as funny/serious, sad/happy, good/bad, selfish/unselfish, scared/brave, trusting/questioning) being co-opted by the other or losing its vibrancy. In other words, the characteristics of <u>funny</u> and the characteristics of <u>serious</u> are **both** present **and** equally experienced in and by the person.

The domestication process teaches us an "either this **or** that" mindset. Often, as children we heard it in the form of the adult admonishing: "Do what I say **or** you are a bad child." This either/or mindset is a reflection of a distorted sacral chakra. For those of us who have experienced psychological counseling, we may have encountered this balancing of opposites in the therapist proposing: "Let's consider that you do not have to choose **either** this **or** that. Instead, you can choose **both** this **and** that." It is truly a mind-boggling concept when first encountered because suddenly a whole new way of perceiving life's choices opens up.

A clear and balanced sacral chakra powers the experience of the natural mammal: playful and innocent, powerful and vulnerable, and capable and needy. Through the sacral chakra, the information linked with ordinary or material creativity is processed and materialized. The most obvious is the creation of a child out of the energies of ovum and sperm. But others abound: gardens, paintings, crafts are just a few examples. This creative force also contributes energy for solving ordinary problems.

When we enlist the Need-Help-Action triangle, we are inviting the energies of the sacral chakra into our healing. We are bringing the energies of the sacral chakra to create something new into the physical realms of our lives. We therefore have the supportive energies to create an action that creates a change. These sacral energies provide the means for restoring the awareness of our needs and vulnerabilities as well as capabilities and strengths so that we can act in ways that care for those needs. We can act and do something that changes our lives now.

Let's now apply the First Turn to yours and Josephine's Drama Dances.

How to Use Need-Help-Action Triangle for Healing

2. REPEAT the Six-Pointed Star Meditation.

3. IDENTIFY THE NEED. When we step onto the Drama Dance (DD) floor, what need are we trying to meet? The DD is a distortion in the root chakra, which we are trying to heal. Therefore, we look to the information about the root chakra to discover the need. (See pages 44-45) When the root chakra is healthy, we experience ourselves as strong, protected, plugged-in, safe, secure, alive, vital, and with a sure trust in our own abilities and in our environment. It is the base that lays the foundation for knowing ourselves as powerful. The answer to the question is always something to do with safety, survival, security, trust, and vitality.

What is your need? Safety, survival, security, trust, and vitality?

When Josephine is asked this question, she answers: "Survival. I am just barely making it through these days dealing with my mother dying, my father in a nursing home and being responsible for doing something with all their things. I spend my days picking up one item to do something with it and before I know it I am knee-deep in tears."

4. IDENTIFY THE HELP. Examine what help is required to meet the identified need. Survival is a basic need and involves the survival of our whole selves. When we ask what help do we require for meeting this need, the answer is chosen from three transformational qualities: self-love, forgiveness or truth. Please read pages 103-109 for a full description of the qualities in regards to energetic information, descriptions and their use of this healing process.

What is the help? Self-love? Forgiveness? Truth?

Josephine quickly replies: "Forgiveness". A look of surprise flashes across her face as if she had no idea that forgiveness had anything to do with this situation.

5. IDENTIFY THE ACTION. Ask what action is needed to meet the identified need with the help of the identified quality.

Josephine, what action do you choose to take to meet your need for survival? You have forgiveness as a quality to help you.

"Drop the superwoman act." It is out of her mouth before she realizes she even had the thought.

6. CHOOSE A WORD OR SENTENCE that encapsulates your answers. Use the NHA drawing to record this information. This will help magnify the information related to the need, help, and action. As a guide, look at Josephine's answers diagrammed below.

Pointers

1. When asking and answering the questions, usually the first thought is the right and best answer. Avoid second guessing yourself and go with the first thought. Research and background information on this process can be found in the chapter titled "Quick! What's your first thought?" on pages 161-163.

2. With this information in hand, we may be tempted to dig deeper and talk more and at great length about this information. This would be the usual method in most counseling approaches. What happens—way too often—when we explore the meanings and stories around the drama information, is a return to the drama triangle. If we start to put specifics to how Josephine will actually "Drop the superwoman act," Josephine will usually return to the Drama. Persecutor statements such as "You think you are so great—that you can do everything better than anyone else" proliferate. It is similar to taking a right turn when going straight ahead will get you to your destination in less time and using less energy. Going straight ahead will also prevent the kindling[49] of re-experiencing original trauma involved in this drama dance.

---

[49] For more descriptions on kindling, see pages 68-69.

3. Whenever we find ourselves slipping back into the Drama, doing any of the energetic healing techniques, especially the Six-Pointed Star Meditation will support us staying off the DD floor. See pages 117-132.

Let's diagram Josephine's answers on the NEED-HELP-ACTION drawing.

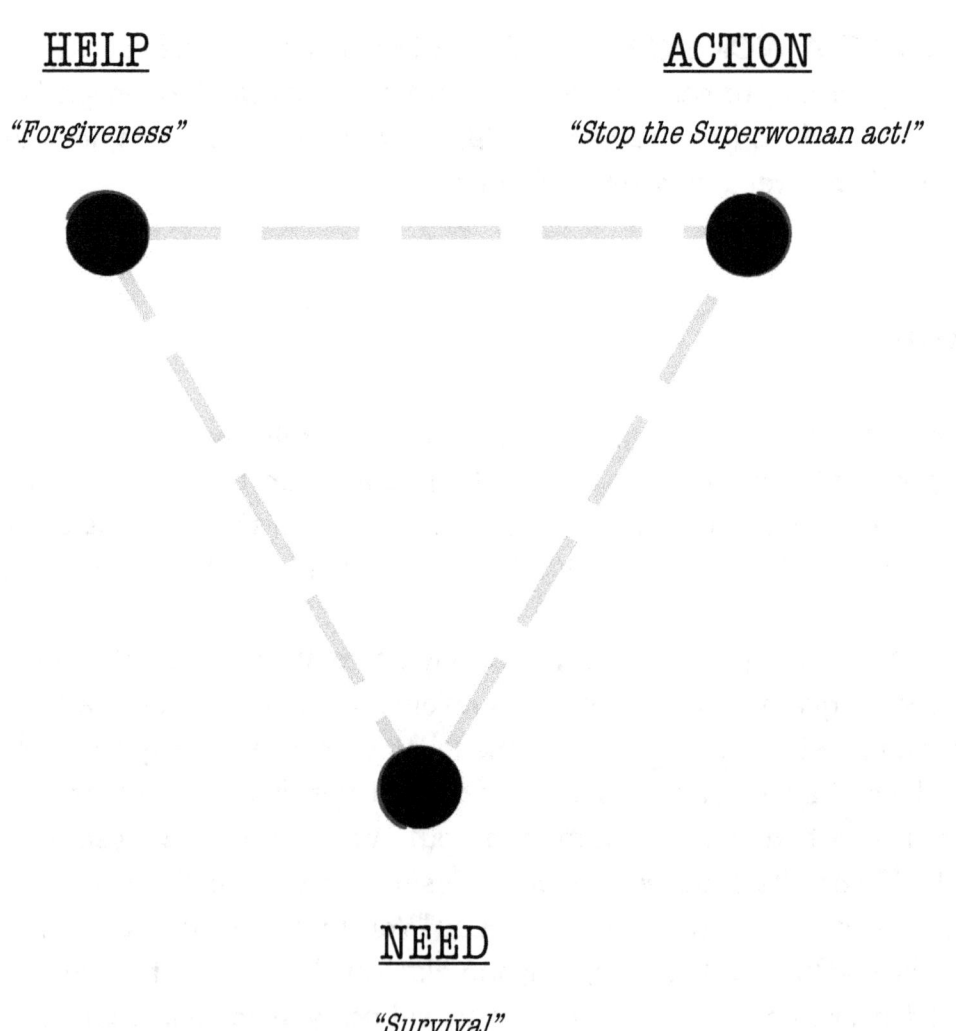

Review and Summary of First Turn

Three Turns of a Kaleidoscope: Healing The Victim Within

PREP ONE
  Do the Six-Pointed Star Meditation.
PREP TWO
  Identify one Natural Mammal Triangle experience in your own life.
PREP THREE
  Choose one Drama Dance experience in your own life.

FIRST TURN
  1. Complete the Need-Action-Help Triangle drawing. Then,
  2. Repeat the Six-Pointed Star Meditation. Next, we
  3. Use our Drama experience and answered the questions:
     - Identify the Need. When we step onto the Drama Dance (DD) floor, what need are we trying to meet? The answer to the question is always something to do with safety, survival, security, trust, and vitality.
     - Identify the Help. Examine what help is required to meet the identified need. Choose from three transformational qualities: self-love, forgiveness or truth.
     - Identify the Action. Ask what action is needed to meet the identified need with help of the identified quality.
  4. Choose a word or sentence that encapsulated your answers.
  5. Record this information on the NHA drawing
  6. Experience an energetic healing technique.

Now on to the SECOND TURN and the second healing triangle!

NOTES:

Second Turn

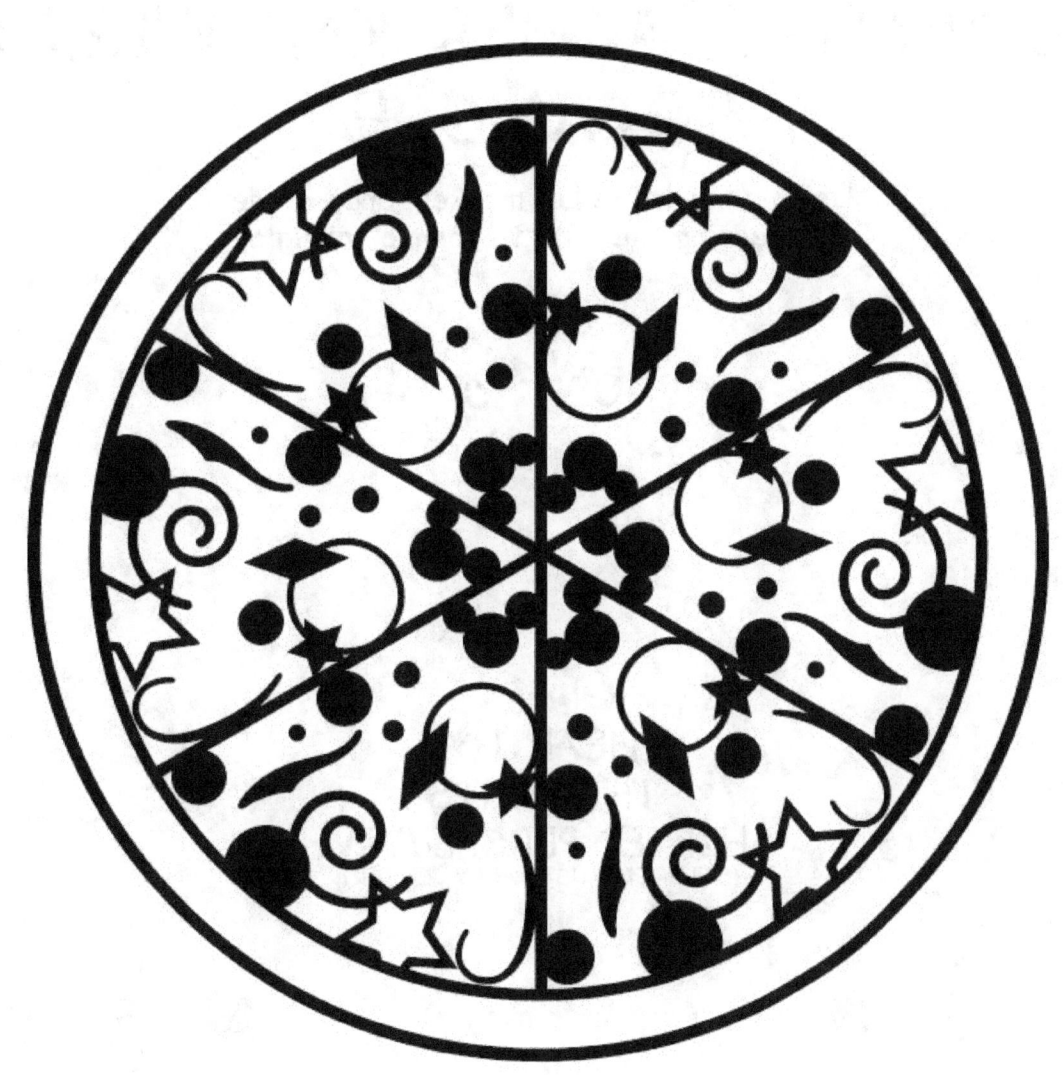

STUDENT-TEACHER-KNOWLEDGE TRIANGLE

Using a bright yellow marker, draw a line connecting the dots to form a triangle

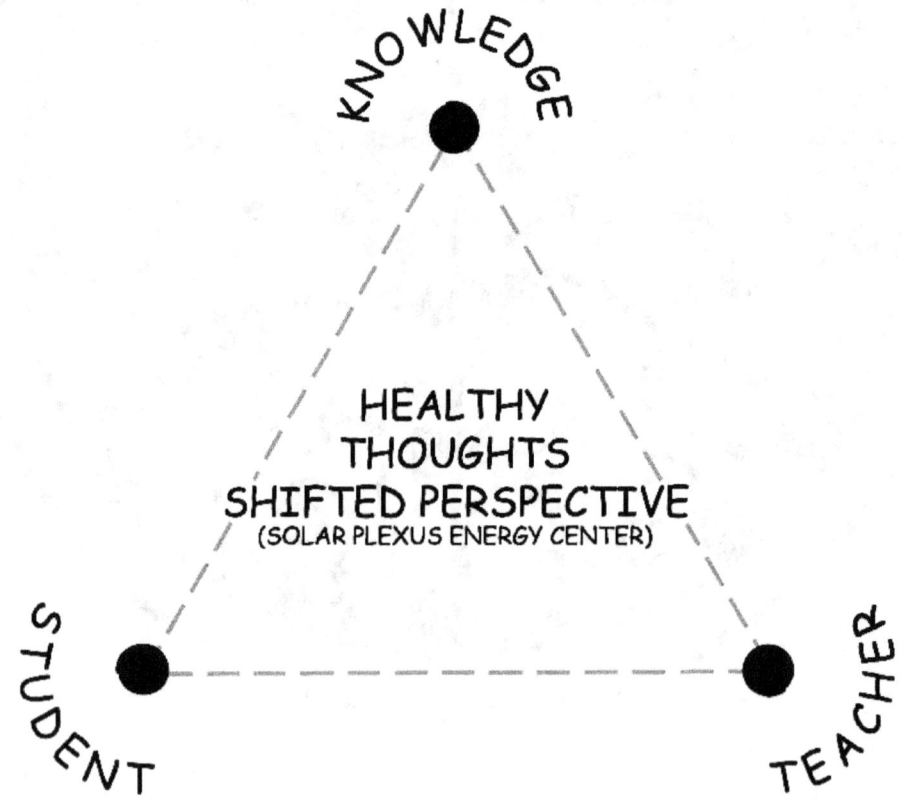

Second Turn:
Shifting Awareness to Learning

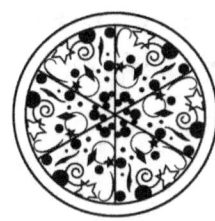

> ### SECOND TURN
>
> - Complete or Trace the drawing of the Student-Teacher-Knowledge Triangle.
> - Repeat Six-Pointed Star Meditation.
> - Using your Drama experience:
>   Identify the Student by asking, "Who is the Student?"
>   Identify the Teacher by asking, "Who is the Teacher?"
>   Discover the Knowledge by asking, "What am I learning from the teacher when I dance this drama?"
> - Choose a word or sentence that encapsulates your answers.
> - Record this information on the STK drawing
> - Experience an energetic healing technique as needed.

The Student-Teacher-Knowledge Triangle is the second turn of the kaleidoscope and the second of the three healing triangles. (See page 75 for diagram of all three triangles.) Notice that the drawing of the Student-Teacher-Knowledge Triangle depicts this shape from a different direction. The previously downward tip of previous triangles is now pointing upward, suggesting a movement toward higher spiritual energies and perception.

Imagine again looking through that new, beautifully made, kaleidoscope. Now envision yourself turning the dial until a new pattern appears. This pattern is a reflection of the second of the three mirrors inside the kaleidoscope. It provides a shift in perspective from meeting basic needs of trust and safety to learning from the school of the Three-Stepping Drama Dance.

This second triangular-shaped mirror helps us to gain insight into harmful thoughts and beliefs. Through the Student-Teacher-Knowledge refraction, we can perceive with increased self-awareness. Here, we open to learning and connecting to the information gleaned from the Drama Dance experience.

We begin the Second Turn by 1. Completing the Student-Teacher-Knowledge triangle. By using the color yellow, we invite the energetic vibrations that increase mental clarity and personal power to act for our welfare.

Student-Teacher-Knowledge Triangle through the Eyes of the Human Energy System

The Student-Teacher-Knowledge healing triangle is associated with the energy of the third chakra: the solar plexus energy center, located at the level of the upper abdomen, just below the diaphragm, and middle back.

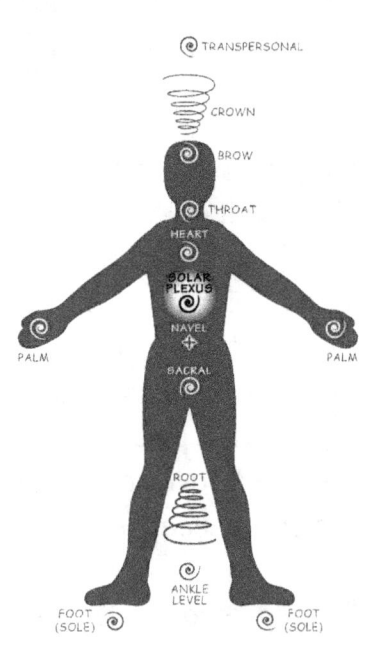

This chakra processes energetic information that is related to ordinary thoughts, to digesting information, and to self-esteem and personal power. The energy of this chakra manifests in empowering us to stand up for ourselves and to process more complex information than danger, threats or emotions. The processing of information at the vibrational level of the solar plexus chakra allows us to add, subtract, plan and execute simple projects. It powers what we think and comprehend.

These many thoughts and beliefs are all encoded in the energetic threads of this center. The encoding is like bits of energy—like computer bytes or subatomic particles—that when put together in a certain way conveys a specific message. The more we think a thought or espouse a belief, the more energy is infused into that construction. The more energy, the more it persists as constructed. Some thoughts are helpful, clear, straight, and true. Some are hurtful, distorted, crooked and false.

If I have a thought such as "I am the only person who can get anything done right" that I tell to myself repeatedly, the thought is strongly energized. Therefore it powers much of the way I live and relate to others and to myself. Since the thought is not true and is distorted, my perceptions are skewed.

One way to change this situation is by de-constructing the thought. That is: take apart the building blocks of the thought and construct a new thought. Because thoughts are more subtle (faster) energy than things, this is easier to do than de-constructing a Lego block creation! The powerful healing energies harnessed through the second turn and the second triangle assist in the deconstruction of distorted thoughts.

We often are unaware of the thoughts that power our daily living. This is particularly so when we are immersed in the Drama Dance. The Student-Teacher-Knowledge Triangle helps us access strongly energized thoughts that start and keep the Drama Dance in motion.

Pointers

This second healing triangular process is often more challenging than the first. We are getting below the surface, down beyond where the Drama Dance boldly keeps us. To help, we employ the transformational qualities of Compassion, Wisdom and Higher Purpose. These qualities are associated with the energy center in and around the brow.

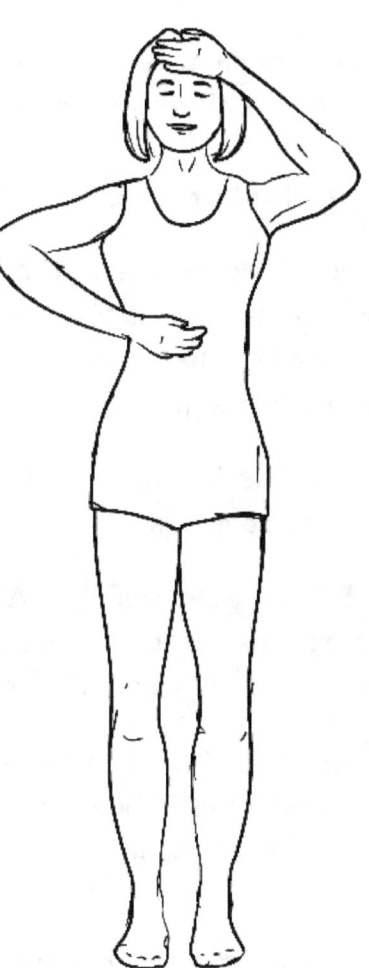

If you find yourself desiring to fling yourself back on the DD floor, stop! Move your attention to your breathing and just watch yourself breathe for a minute. Then, place one hand on your Solar Plexus and one on your Brow. Allow the Universal Healing Energies to infuse through your hands and into the two chakras. Let yourself become aware of which quality—Compassion, Wisdom or Higher Purpose—will help you now. Then call on the chosen quality to help answer the Second Turn questions. See pages 103-104, 110-114 for more information about these transformational qualities.

How to Use Student-Teacher-Knowledge Triangle

2. REPEAT the Six-Pointed Star Meditation.

3. IDENTIFY THE STUDENT by asking, "Who is the Student?"

In each Drama Dance, there is a student disguised as one of the VRP roles.

Start by asking yourself, in your Drama Dance, who is the Student?

The most obvious answer is: "I am." Right! However, sometimes the answer will be someone or something else. If so, allow the first thought answer to be honored and follow the emerging process.

Josephine, who is the student in your Drama Dance? "Oh, I definitely am! The part of me that was whining about needing rest"

4. IDENTIFY THE TEACHER by asking, "Who is the Teacher?"

In each Drama Dance, the teacher is often camouflaged in the role of the Persecutor or suggested in the answer to "What is the action that will meet the need?" The teacher can be an aspect of you, a thing, a situation, or another person.

Who is the teacher, Josephine? "The voice inside of me that said I have no right to complain."

5. DISCOVER THE KNOWLEDGE by asking, "What am I learning from the teacher when I dance this drama?" Again, the first thought in response to the question is usually the thought to follow.

Josephine, what are you learning from the voice in your head? Josephine answers: "That I believe I have to do everything, that no one else can do it right. That I believe I can't take time for myself or the whole world will fall apart."

6. CHOOSE A WORD OR SENTENCE that encapsulates your answers. Use the STK drawing to record this information. This will help magnify and clarify the information. As a guide, look at Josephine's answers diagrammed below.

Let's diagram Josephine's answers on the Student-Teacher-Knowledge drawing.

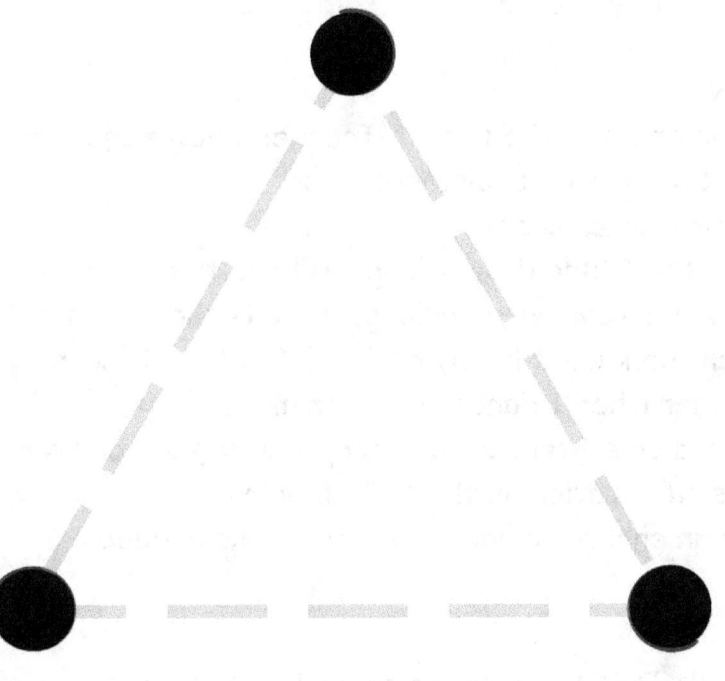

KNOWLEDGE

"That I believe I have to do everything, that no one else can do it right. That I believe I can't take time for myself or the whole world will fall apart."

STUDENT

"Oh, I definitely am! The part of me that was whining about getting rest."

TEACHER

"The voice inside of me that said I have no right to complain."

Review and Summary of the Second Turn

Three Turns of a Kaleidoscope: Healing The Victim Within

PREP ONE
   Do the Six-Pointed Star Meditation.
PREP TWO
  Identify one Natural Mammal Triangle experience in your own life.
PREP THREE
  Choose one Drama Dance experience in your own life.
FIRST TURN
  Using your Drama experience: identify the need, help and action.

SECOND TURN
  1. Complete the drawing of Student-Teacher-Knowledge Triangle.
  2. Repeat the Six-Pointed Star Meditation.
  3. In your Drama experiences,
      - Identify the Student by asking, "Who is the Student?"
      - Identify the Teacher by asking, "Who is the Teacher?"
      - Discover the Knowledge by asking, "What am I learning from the teacher when I dance this drama?"
  4. Choose a word or sentence that encapsulated your answers.
  5. Record this information on the STK drawing
  6. Experience an energetic healing technique as needed.

On to the THIRD TURN and the third healing triangle!

Third Turn

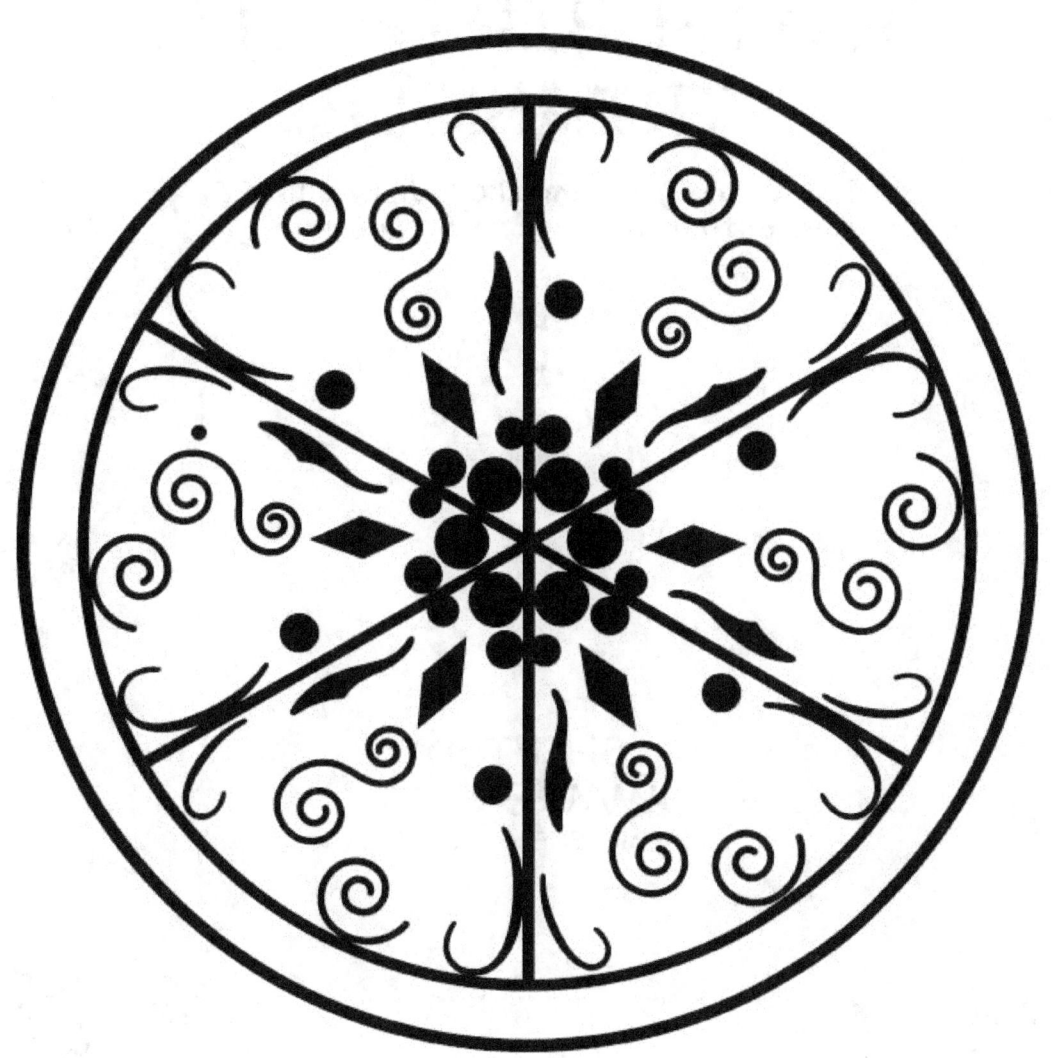

DEATH-BIRTH-LIFE TRIANGLE

Using a green marker, draw a line connecting the dots to form a triangle

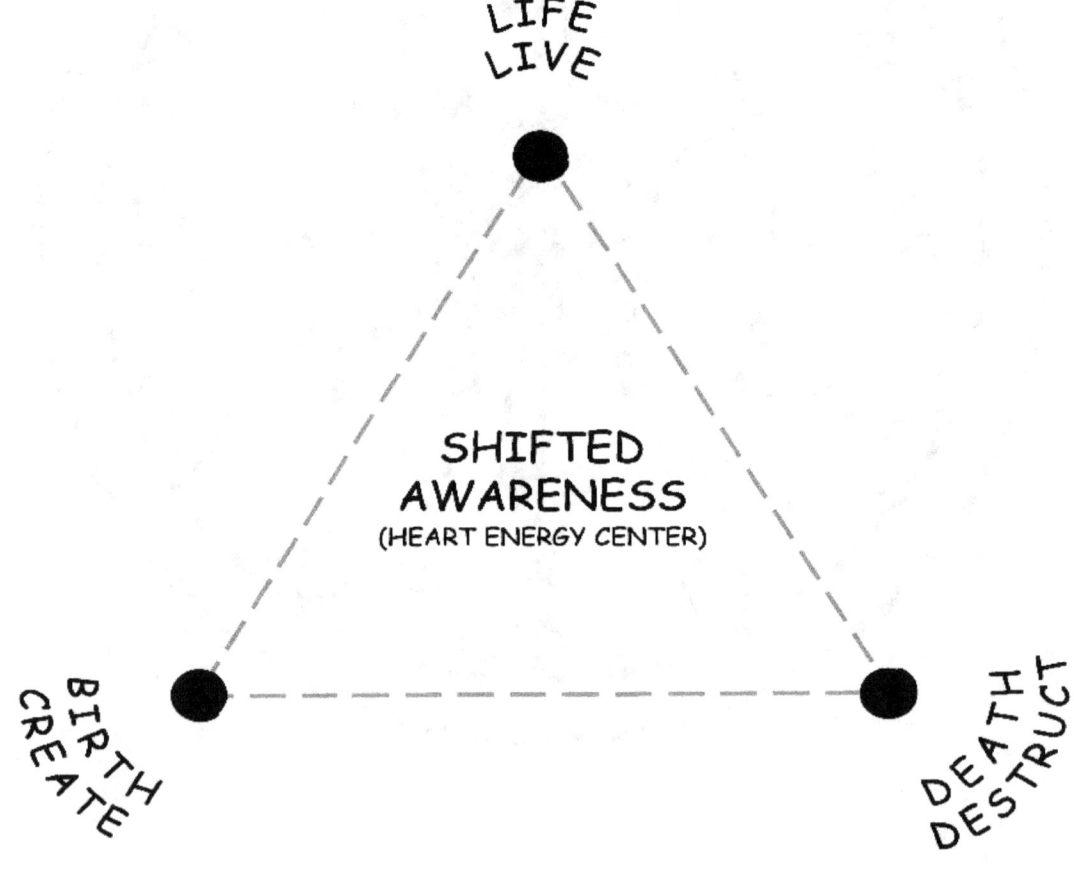

Third Turn: Transforming to Living Anew

> **THIRD TURN**
>
> ✁ Complete or Trace the Death-Birth-Life Triangle drawing.
>
> ✁ Repeat the Six-Pointed Star Meditation.
>
> ✁ Using your Drama experience
>
>   Identify the Death by asking, "What in me needs to or is ready to die or de-struct?"
>
>   Identify the Birth by asking, "What in me, is ready to be created?"
>
>   Reap the Living by asking, "What will that look like in my actual day to day life?"
>
> ✁ Reinforce the New: place one hand on your Heart Chakra and one on your Crown. Allow the Universal Healing Energies to infuse through your hands and into the two chakras. Allow Self-Love, Forgiveness, Truth, Compassion, Wisdom and Higher Purpose to fill your heart and the new awareness.
>
> ✁ Choose a word or sentence that encapsulates your answers. Record this information on the DBL drawing

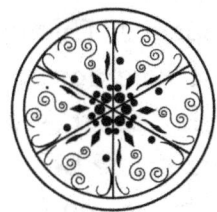

We begin the Third Turn by
1. Completing the Death-Birth-Life Triangle on the opposite page. We use the color green because this is the color associated with the energetic vibrations of healing transformation.

The Death-Birth-Life Triangle is the third turn of the kaleidoscope and the last of the three healing triangles. Notice that the drawing of this triangle, like the Student-Teacher-Knowledge Triangle, orients with the apex pointing upward. This symbolizes a movement into higher states of awareness and faster energetic dimensions. Einstein is quoted frequently as saying that a problem cannot be solved at the level at which it was created. This is true for the Drama Dance. To solve and heal the energetic configurations that we experience as the drama dance, we must leave the root chakra energies and climb up the chakra pole. So far, we have shinnied up into and through the sacral and solar plexus and have arrived at the heart level.

From the heart level, let's discover the view through the kaleidoscope. Imagine again that you are looking through that new, beautifully made, kaleidoscope. Now, envision yourself turning the dial until a new pattern appears. This pattern is a reflection of the third of the three mirrors inside the kaleidoscope. This third triangular-shaped mirror, Death-Birth-Life, helps destroy or de-struct, in order that something new can be created. Life, the space between birth and death, is a constant flow between creation and destruction for renewal or restoration. It provides a shift in perspective from meeting basic needs of trust and safety in the first turn, to learning from the school of Three-Stepping Drama Dance in the second turn, to the alchemical realm of transformation in the third turn. This transformation moves us from the physical into the spiritual realms.

Death-Birth-Life Triangle
through the Eyes of the Human Energy System

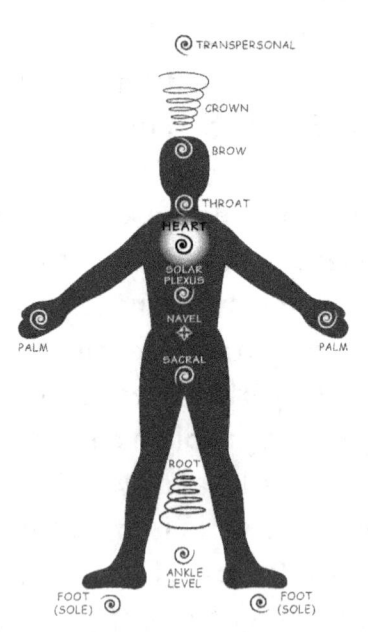

The Death-Birth-Life healing triangle is associated with the energy of the fourth chakra: the heart energy center, located at the level of the middle chest and mid-section of the upper back. This chakra processes energetic information that is related to receiving love. Through the heart chakra we take in the Universal Energies that vibrate at a frequency we describe as love. The heart chakra is considered the chakra of transformation. Likened to an electrical transformer station, the heart chakra transforms the energies of the lower (slower frequencies) chakras to the upper (faster) chakras. This means that the energetic information of the root (safety and vitality), sacral (ordinary emotions) and solar plexus (ordinary thoughts) are transformed in the heart (unconditional love and acceptance) to be lived out in the higher realms of the throat (living one's truth), brow (perceiving clearly and with discernment) and crown (oneness). The flow of energy through the chakras also occurs from crown, through brow, through throat, then transformed in heart, to materialize in the ordinary world. Therefore the heart chakra energies can take a skewed belief like "I am too scared to lead groups" and transform that belief into a totally new awareness.

The sages of Vedic India "would point out that the real shift is one of allegiance. When we die we give up allegiance to 'consciousness filled with physical objects' to 'consciousness filled with subtle objects'." [50] Yet, this shift in allegiance also occurs when an old way dies. We give up our faithfulness to a consciousness filled with the constructs, perspectives, thoughts, and beliefs of that old way. For example, when I gave up the belief that I was too scared to be a group leader, I gave up my commitment to that view of myself. I stepped into another world in which I viewed myself as brave enough to learn how to be a group leader. My loyalty changed with how I viewed myself with this new consciousness. I still may experience fear in leading a group but I am no longer **too** scared. Through the Death-Birth-Life refraction, one can move from helpless to safe to self-aware to a completely new awareness. Out of this transformation, we live our life anew.

How to Use Death-Birth-Life Triangle for Healing

2. REPEAT the Six-Pointed Star Meditation.

3. IDENTIFY THE DEATH by asking, "What in me needs to or is ready to die or de-struct?"

Recall or re-read the answers you recorded on VRP, NHA and STK diagrams. What is the knowledge that relates to the need or action that arose out of your drama dance? Then ask yourself, in your Drama Dance "What needs to or is ready to die or de-struct?"

Imagine that what needs to be destructed is made out of Lego blocks or knitted yarn or clay. You can destruct it as easily as taking the blocks apart, unraveling the yarn or kneading the clay. Usually the answer relates to what you have or are learning, that is, the knowledge you identified. Often it is a distorted or false idea or belief.

---
50 Deepak Chopra p. 130

Allow the first thought answer to be honored and follow the emerging process.

Josephine, What needs to or is ready to die or de-struct in your Drama Dance?

Josephine answers: "That I have to be superwoman all the time; that only I can do anything right"

4. IDENTIFY THE BIRTH by asking, "What, in me, is ready to be created?"

Out of the de-structed, something can be born or newly created. So the idea: "That I have to be superwoman all the time; that only I can do anything right" is taken apart and re-constructed. What is created? What is birthed out of the Lego blocks, the unraveled yarn or the lump of clay?

"What, in you, is ready to be re-created, Josephine?" "I can rest when I need to!"

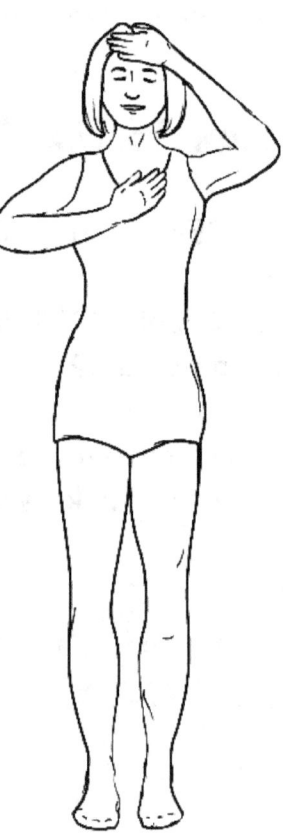

5. REAP THE LIVING by asking, "What will that look like in your actual day to day life?" Again, the first thought in response to the question is usually the thought to follow. "Cat naps. I used to love to take catnaps. Just sort of doze off for a few minutes. For years, whenever I would doze off during the day, I would scold myself. Not any more! (Josephine asserted with a strong commitment to self.)

6. REINFORCE THE NEW: place one hand on your Heart Chakra and one on your Crown. Allow the Universal Healing Energies to infuse through your hands and into the two chakras. Allow Compassion, Wisdom and Higher Purpose to fill your heart and the new awareness.

7. CHOOSE a word or sentence that encapsulates your answers. Use the DBL drawing to record this information. Look at the diagram of Josephine's answers to guide you in answering and recording yours.

Let's diagram Josephine's answers on the Death-Birth-Life drawing.

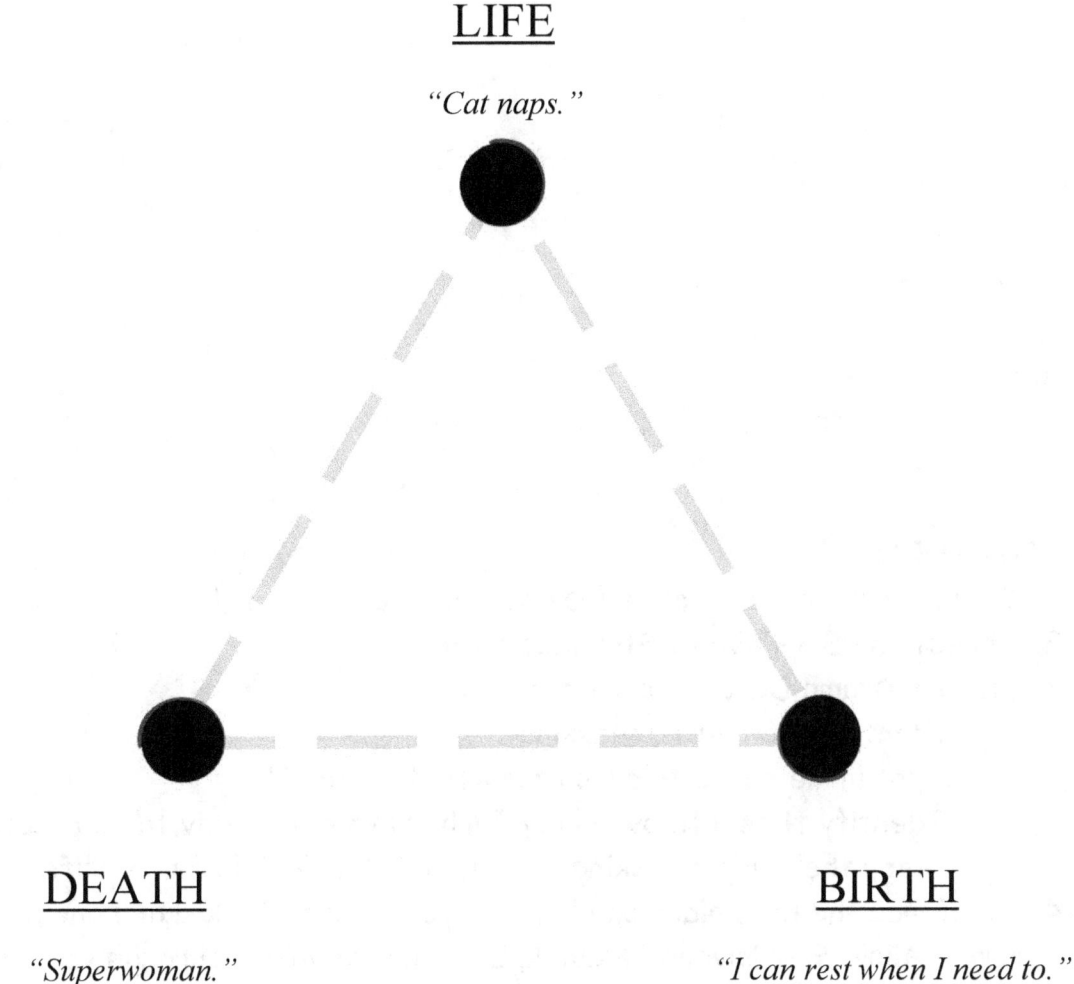

After doing this process, sit or move in an intentional way that allows you to quietly be with yourself. Even better, go play! Avoid the temptation to dig deeper into the information. Allow (that means avoid pushing, forcing, digging, explaining, making happen, working at) the healing energies, which have been activated by the turning of the Kaleidoscope, to be alive and active within you.

Review and Summary of Third Turn

Three Turns of a Kaleidoscope: Healing The Victim Within

PREP ONE
  Do the Six-Pointed Star Meditation.
PREP TWO
  Identify one Natural Mammal Triangle experience in your own life.
PREP THREE
  Choose one Drama Dance experience in your own life.
FIRST TURN
  Using your Drama experience: identify the need, help and action.
SECOND TURN
  Using your Drama experience: identify the student and teacher and discover the knowledge.

THIRD TURN
1. Complete the drawing of the Death-Birth-Life Triangle.
2. Repeat the Six-Pointed Star Meditation.
3. In your Drama Dance experience:
    - Identify the death by asking, "What in me needs to or is ready to destruct?"
    - Identify the birth by asking, "What in me, is ready to be created?"
    - Reap the living by asking, "What will that look like in my life?"
4. Reinforce the new: place one hand on your Heart Chakra and one on your Crown. Allow the Universal Healing Energies to infuse through your hands and into the two chakras. This allows Self-Love, Truth, Forgiveness, Compassion, Wisdom and Higher Purpose to fill your heart and the new awareness.
5. Choose a word or sentence that encapsulated our answers.
6. Record this information on the DBL drawing.

Now Celebrate!

Next are the in-depth descriptions of the six spiritual qualities as helpers in healing the Victim within.

Six Spiritual Qualities

As described in Part One, the healing vibrations—necessary for healing the Victim within—are subtle spiritual energies. The two helping triangles, which interweave to form the six-pointed star, depict the energetic blueprint through which these powerful energies flow. We accessed these energies blended into wholeness when we traced the diagram of the six-pointed star and did the six-pointed star meditation. In this chapter, we will focus on accessing the energies of the individual qualities of Self-Love, Forgiveness, Truth, Compassion, Wisdom, and Higher Purpose.

First complete the diagrams of the two triangles on the next page. We use the color sky blue and indigo because these are the colors associated with the energetic vibrations of throat and brow chakras respectively. Recall that the energies of the fifth or throat chakra support and power the triangle of Truth-Self Love-Forgiveness and the energies of the sixth or brow energy center sustain the triangle of Compassion-Wisdom-Higher Purpose. The completion of these triangles—as with the prior triangles—creates healing connections within our memories, bodies, and brains.

In addition to tracing the diagrams of these helping triangles, we can access the spiritual energies by 1. Asking for the help of the qualities, by
2. Employing the healing technique: the Chakra Correspondence and by
3. Studying the meaning and knowledge of the qualities and applying this intelligence.

1. The easiest way to access the spiritual energies is simply to invoke the essence of one of the qualities, allowing the energies of the qualities to assist in the healing the Victim within. When we ask, "What is the help to meet this need in this particular Drama Dance?" we may answer truth. Simply, ask for truth to help in meeting this need. In this method, the intellectual or expressive understandings of the qualities are not necessary.

2. Another method for accessing the six spiritual qualities is the hands-on energetic healing practice: the Chakra Correspondence described on page 125. The hands are used to connect the flow of the energies from the throat

and brow chakras to the chakras associated with the Drama Dance and the Three Turns (root, sacral, solar plexus and heart).

3. To gain a deeper knowledge of the qualities, study the descriptions that follow, then apply this intelligence to the healing process. For example, one of the descriptors is "Truth is telling it like it is." Maybe, this descriptor clicks with you or resonates or increases a sense of peace or fits your situation. "Telling it like it is" to yourself may become the action for meeting the need of safety.

In the following sections, each of the qualities is described in detail, including quotes from philosophers, spiritual teachers, world leaders, healers and writers. Each description has a Sacred Feminine image, an object and an animal that personifies the quality. Some descriptions include personal memoirs.

Truth/Self-Love/ Forgiveness Triangle
Using a sky-blue marker, draw a line connecting the dots to form a triangle.

Compassion/Wisdom/ Higher Purpose Triangle
Using an indigo marker, draw a line connecting the dots to form a triangle.

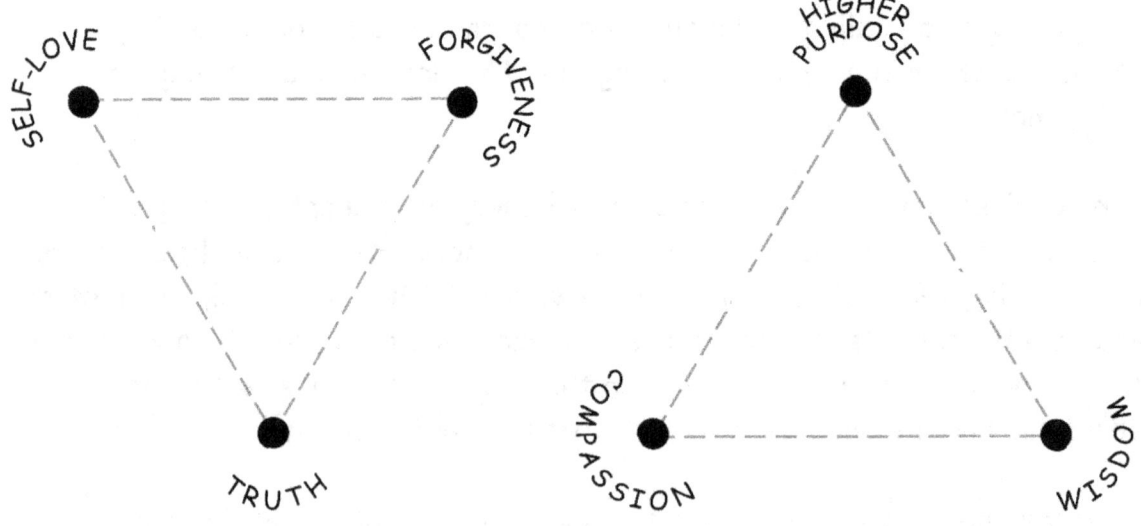

Truth

Sacred Feminine: Tara, Hindu and Celtic Goddess: "She Who Brings Forth Life, She Who Is The Embodiment Of Wisdom, The Great Compassionate Mother, The Star Of Heaven"
Object: plumb line, deep bowl
Animal: Eagle

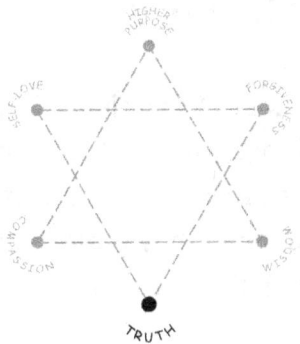

"Truth is layered like an onion or an artichoke. So the task of becoming free is akin to peeling away layers of truth, like the leaves of an artichoke, to uncover the core truth that transforms experience. Core truths always transform experience and always have to do with oneself, never with one's upbringing or what anyone else says or does, past or present. Core truths always evolve from profound self-acceptance."   Roberta Jean Bryant

Truth is telling it like it is.

Truth is the Divine expressing Itself. When we speak or act the truth, the Divine is expressing Itself through our individual being.

Musician and therapist Tom Kenyon tells this story on the CD[51] I'm listening to as I prepare lunch. He has a set of seven crystal bowls specially made by lamas in Tibet. He is quite attached to these bowls for they produce incredibly pure tones when touched. One day, a child breaks his favorite bowl. He plays the largest bowl and a pure tone is evoked. As I listen, the bowl and I synchronize. I attune to the bowl's vibration and feel the rightness of the tone within me. Then Kenyon strikes the broken bowl; I shudder. The tone is so discordant; I want to run away from it. My body knows truth by its ability to detect a vibration that sits well with it.

Truth is something we know with our whole being; it attunes us and we cannot be dissuaded. Truth sits well with and in our bodies. Truth produces an ease that allows us to swallow smoothly, to breathe deeply, to see clearly, to hear acutely, to smell sharply, to taste discriminately, to move effortlessly and to know unequivocally.

---

[51] Tom Kenyon "The Ghandarva Ceremony: History and Context" CD Track 1

Self-Love

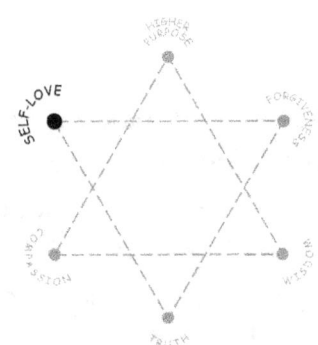

Sacred Feminine: Oshun, the West African goddess of love, art and sensuality who is "the place where the river waters meet the ocean"[52]
Object: shawl, blanket
Animal: Orangutan

Self-Love is caring for oneself. In *Care Of The Soul*, Thomas Moore asserts, loud and clear, that the soul is not to be understood but cared for.

Self-Love is self-acceptance and forgiveness of oneself. It is giving up toxic guilt, shame and self-hatred.

In the online encyclopedia, *Wikipedia*[53], love is described as "a basic dimension of human experience that is variously conveyed as a sense of tender affection, an intense attraction, the foundation of intimacy and good interpersonal chemistry, willing self-sacrifice on behalf of another, and as an ineffable sense of affinity or connection to nature, other living beings, or even that which is unseen."

Can we possibly apply all this to ourselves? Will we be tender and affectionate with ourselves? Do we notice a chemistry that sparks as we spend time with our own selves? Are we willing to sacrifice on behalf of self?

The triangular theory of love characterizes love in an interpersonal relationship on three different scales: intimacy, passion, and commitment. According to the author of the theory, psychologist Robert Sternberg, a relationship based on two or more of the above elements is more likely to survive than a relationships based on only one.[54] In the intrapersonal relationship with self, how many elements are present? Do we express intimacy (genuine revealing and receiving of whole self), passion and commitment?

---

52 www.moonlitriver.com/Oshun
53 www.Wikipedia.org
54 www.Wikipedia.org

In my case, commitment was a sticky point in loving myself. Over time I began to realize that commitment means standing with and by my self through "thick and thin". It clearly requires abandoning any abandonment of my self. Notice how this reveals itself in my dreams.

Memoirs Summer 2004, Awake Dreams: "I walk into a large house, down a flight of stairs to the basement. A door at one end of the basement opens to a stone-lined cellar. Everything is a dusty gray. On the walls are hanging emaciated, dirty, smelly people. They are full of weeping wounds and look as if their last breath was a long time ago. Yet I can see that they are still breathing. Their eyes find mine and beseech. I turn my head, avert my eyes and in my mind stomp my foot and say, 'No! I will not take care of them. I won't! Look at them! They should just be put out of their misery.' I turn to an Invisible Being and cry: 'And You! You want me to take care of them!'"

By this time in my life, I have cared for so many others. I have even cared for myself. In fact, I have been practicing self-love for years. However, the above dream has brought the truly unlovable, repulsive, too needy aspects of myself to my attention, a sort of "right in my face" dream. Yet I know I am being called to care for the unlovable and untouchable because I turn to that Greater Self, represented as an Invisible Being, and rail against this calling. Jungian Analyst and Dream expert Marion Woodman relates that our abandoned inner child often turns up in our dreams in a basement below the basement and in terrible shape: dirty and disheveled.

Six weeks later, this awake dream occurs: "I opened a door to a room in which I could only see bodies that had large, deep, bleeding, raw wounds. I saw myself enter the room and care for the wounds, one at a time, by washing, soothing, bandaging. I watched myself care for the wounds in the loving and gentle way I do for others. I knew that these were my wounds from the present time and I cried with joy that I am caring for me." In spite of the railing and refusal – or maybe because of it – I answer the call to care – to love self – not just with words, but also with actions that go deep within me.

Forgiveness

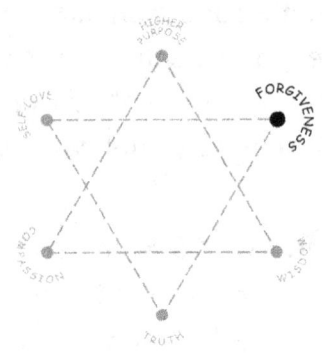

Sacred Feminine: Mary Magdalena
Object: knife or sword
Animal: Dog

Forgiveness is a letting go primarily of shame, blame and a locked-in skewed perception.

Forgiveness is giving up the need for revenge. Chris Faulconer

Forgiveness frees us from our self-imposed virtual prison. It opens the door through which we step out into the home of our true selves.

Forgiveness is the answer to the child's dream of a miracle by which what is broken is made whole again, what is soiled is again made clean.
Dag Hammarskjöld

Forgiveness is the mental, emotional and/or spiritual process of ceasing to feel resentment or anger against another person for a perceived offence, difference or mistake, or ceasing to demand punishment or restitution.[55]

Forgiveness does not change the past, but it does enlarge the future
Paul Boese

Forgiveness is the fragrance the violet sheds on the heel that has crushed it.
Mark Twain

Memoirs Spring 2007 Walking at Radnor Lake on an evening after an all day soft rain, my feet fall on the soggy and misty path. I have left my computer in the middle of writing about forgiveness. "What about you?" I ask myself, "What do you have to say about forgiveness?" Rich, my late husband, comes to my mind. We had so many discussions about forgiveness, for he often said he just couldn't forgive. I used to marvel that he even thought that about himself for he seemed to be the most forgiving of all people. Over our many

---

[55] www.Wikipedia.org

years together, I began to notice that Rich had devised a unique system that didn't involve forgiveness. He just never held anything against others so he had nothing to forgive. If someone did something that would have got me hopping mad, the same thing just slid right past and off Rich. He had the uncanny ability to love others as they were.

I, on the other hand, held onto wrongs as if my life depended on it! I had a "bag" I kept my "slights" in and pulled them out whenever I needed them. Rich would say, "You still remember that? That was ten years ago. How long are you going to make me pay for that?" In our discussions, I was the one who knew how to forgive and I could but I seemed to be so much better at faulting than forgiving.

As I wind down the ridge and into the thick forest, a vision of a tall thin girl appears on the trail ahead. She carries a white canvas bag with pull string closure. I ask her who she is. "I carry the slights for you here in this bag." "Well, how many and what have you got in there?" "None, the bag's empty." No resentments, no slights, no holding onto being injured by another? Maybe this Healing-the-Victim-Within is working! I turn back to the girl. "It's time to get rid of that bag. I don't need it anymore and you don't have to carry it for me anymore. Let's think of what to do with the bag."

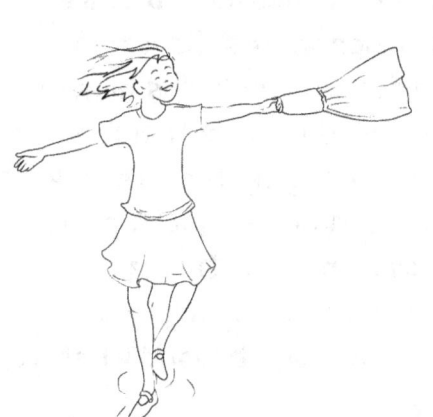

At first the girl is not sure it's a good idea to get rid of the bag. "What will you do with the slights?" I'm perplexed at first but finally realize I just want to continue to let them go. I no longer want to hold onto them. I decide that in the future I will dig a hole in the earth, put any slights in, and cover them over, my own little slight compost pile. I tell her this. Then I ask what she wants to do with the canvas bag. At first she wants to keep it, just in case. I just stand there with her, waiting. Surprisingly, she starts turning in circles, slow at first, then faster. Twirling round and round, she is dancing as free as the wind. The canvas bag, held in her hand, moves with her. She looks so happy. Maybe since she no longer has the job of holding onto my slights and resentments, she can and will dance!

Wisdom

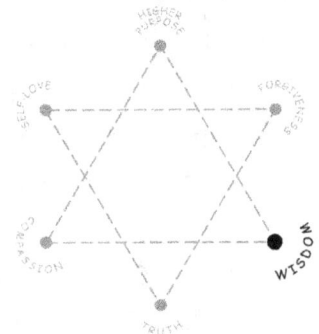

Sacred Feminine: Shekinah (Hebrew word which means "She who dwells". Call on her for comfort, for advise, for blessing, for guidance. She will respond with love and radiating light.)
Object: chalice, lighthouse, beacon, dousing rod
Animal: owl

Wisdom is the ability, developed through experience, insight and reflection, to discern truth and exercise good judgment.[56]

Wisdom is sometimes conceptualized as an especially well-developed form of common sense.

Wisdom is learned by three methods: Reflection (the noblest), imitation (the easiest) and experience (the bitterest).   Confucius

Wisdom is the acquisition "… of practical life experiences — experiences both good and bad. It implies an awareness of both possibilities and limitations, opportunities and barriers, and perhaps especially an awareness of the finitude of life itself."   Robert Scaer

Wisdom is a higher or spiritual awareness that guides our choices and perceptions. It provides a larger Light, which illuminates the whole picture of individual situations and the whole of our lives. As Scaer writes wisdom is acquired thru "practical life experiences" which teach us to seek this higher spiritual knowledge or guidance. It is not merely acquired information from practical life experiences. Wisdom is the act of acknowledging that we lack information and/or direction and are seeking Guidance. When we pick up the quality of Wisdom, we immediately turn toward an awareness of Divine Knowledge and Guidance. We agree to turn away from limited or useless knowledge. We agree to listen to and be guided by Knowledge beyond what we know on an ordinary level.

---

[56] www.Wikipedia.org

Compassion

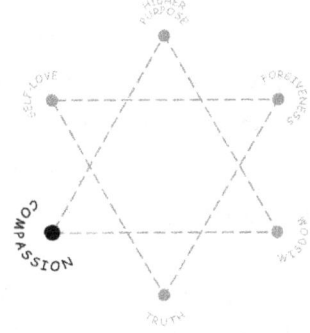

Sacred Feminine: Kwan Yin, Chinese goddess of compassion
Object: begging bowl
Animal: Gorilla

Compassion: "Have you ever been with someone and on listening to their story you became so touched or moved that a tear came to your eyes? Yet at the same time you knew they were suffering...you knew that it would not be helpful to rescue them or try to change them? When we have such an experience, we are in direct contact with our Compassionate Child."
Charles L Whitfield MD

...Compassion like vines climbs anything that stands in the way.   Mark Nepo

Compassion: "When you begin to touch your heart or let your heart be touched, you begin to discover that it's bottomless...that this heart is huge, vast, and limitless. You begin to discover how much warmth and gentleness is there, as well as how much space."
Pema Chodron

Compassion: "We who lived in concentration camps can remember the men who walked through the huts comforting others, giving away their last piece of bread. They may have been few in number, but they offer sufficient proof that everything can be taken from a (hu)man but one thing: the last of the human freedoms—to choose one's attitude in any given set of circumstances, to choose one's own way."
Viktor Frankl

I struggle with this quality. What really is compassion? How is it different from self-love or love? Is it possible to really be compassionate? Am I?
I vividly remember two times in my life when compassion left its mark on me:

Memoirs Spring 1972 My daughters are two years old and I am a single mother. I manage to care for them with a gentle and constant love. I work as a nurse, so we have enough money, just enough. This day, I am sitting on the steps going down to the front door. My partner has just left after we had sat together talking and crying — grieving for the unborn child we created together and whom I aborted the day before. I am still crying, sobbing. My small daughters, with black curls covering their heads and deep brown, almost black eyes, chubby faces, hands, feet, sit down beside me, rest their hands on me and cry with me. They don't say much except "It's okay, Mommy" over and over. They sit with me until the crying subsides and my heart is touched by their quiet acceptance of me as I am.

Spring 1994 It is 2 am. I wake suddenly, full of anxious fear. "Rich, we have to do something. Something's wrong. I can feel it." Our 18-year-old son is in jail – he has been there for three days now. I am sure great harm is happening to him right now. I am inconsolable and Rich has no idea what to do. Distraught, I say: "We have to go down there. We have to check on him." Finally, I say "Call Amy. She will know what to do." Rich calls and Amy (out of a deep sleep and a comfortable bed) comes. She climbs into our bed and holds onto me while I sob and scream and am gripped by a terror for the well being of my "lost" son. I beseech her to do something. Amy says: "Okay, I will." She picks up the phone, dials the city jail, and explains the situation. The person on the other end goes off and checks on our son and comes back to report that our son is sleeping. He is okay. Could this be? I am not sure. However, I am sure that Amy and Rich have wrapped me in the blanket of compassion. They hold me until I am calm and sleepy. That morning I awake and hear myself singing: "This is the day that the Lord has made. Let us rejoice and be glad!" I notice the sun is shining.

I remember my dream of caring for my deeply wounded self and think maybe this is compassion too. This is the act of being with someone as they are and when things are really a mess. When the wounds are full of dirt and pus, when the emotions are ragged and high pitched, when the faces are ugly, the words mean-spirited, the actions threatening, when situations cannot be fixed, yet we sit with each other or with ourselves, and do our best to be present. I look up compassion and companion in the dictionary; seems like they must be related. Compassion: suffering with during distressing situations   Companion: one that accompanies another.

The stories above are of distressing situations. My daughters and Rich and Amy were able to be with me; to be companions during great distress equals compassion. Choosing to use the quality of compassion means that we allow as well as invite others to be with us in the midst of a distressful time.

Higher Purpose

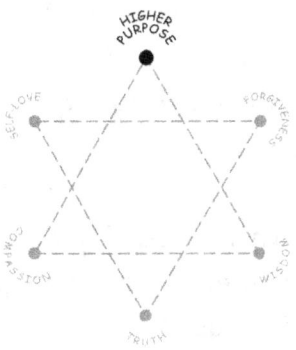

Sacred Feminine: Isis, ancient Egyptian goddess depicted as the Mother of All or the Great Cosmic Mother
Object: hot air balloon
Animal: dolphin

Higher Purpose is the awareness of and living through the lens of deep meaning.
                                                                    Victor Frankl

Higher Purpose is intention for the highest good for oneself and all.

Higher Purpose is heightened awareness. With higher purpose an activity, like walking, takes on deep meaning so that one walks with intention for a greater good. I can walk appreciative of and grateful for the beauty of the sky and trees, the uplifting song of the birds, the invigorating rush of the river water, the soothing coolness of the wind, the strong support of the earth beneath my feet, and the clearing of my tangled emotions and thoughts. I can walk in solidarity and support for causes important to me: breast cancer research, gay and lesbian pride, multiple sclerosis, and affordable housing. I can walk committed to my physical health.

Higher Purpose gives meaning to any and all experiences.

Nurse healer Linda Hunt tells this story: "I am driving down the road when the car in front of me slams on the brakes. Just barely in time, I am able to stop my car without hitting the car in front of me. After I catch my breath, I say to the driver: 'Please be more careful, pay attention, take it easier. Please slow down and give more space and signal when you put on your brakes. This will help you to avoid hurting yourself and others.' My husband looks at me perplexed and asks: 'Is that your way of telling him off for being such a jerk?' 'No, I was talking to him to help him.' My husband is even more perplexed: 'But he can't hear you!' 'Oh, I was talking to his higher self.'"

Linda often takes the moments while driving a car — an ordinary activity — and converts it to a higher purpose. When she drives by a person, she says: "I bless and recognize the Divine Being that you are."

Higher Purpose is a template that we can apply to any and all life situations. With this quality we are able to ask for and invite in higher (faster) spiritual energies. Higher purpose extends a strong and purposeful hand that helps us out of quagmires or situations of limited vision. By grasping that hand, we find ourselves on an elevated hill — solid beneath our feet — from which our view of the terrain of our life is more complete. Before we had walked without direction or had sloshed through or been stuck in the mud. Now, from the higher purpose knoll we see the meandering path and are aware of where that path is leading.

For example, I am in two fender bender auto accidents within one month. I ask the question: "What spiritual guide is trying to get my attention? What is the message I have failed to hear?" The answer? "I am not following spiritual direction." I am stumped. I think I have been doing all that I can humanly do! So I meditate and muse and mull for a few days. I finally realize that I have been given a specific spiritual direction and have not acted on this direction. The Higher Purpose quality takes out the ear plugs and takes off the blindfold and I can now act on the spiritual direction I have received.

Summary

In healing the Victim within, we may access the healing energies of Self-Love, Forgiveness, Truth, Compassion, Wisdom, and Higher Purpose by
1. Tracing the diagram of the six-pointed star and the helping triangles,
2. Doing the six-pointed star meditation,
3. Asking for the help of the qualities,
4. Employing the healing technique: the Chakra Correspondence, and
5. Studying and applying the meaning and knowledge of the qualities.

Part V: RETURN TO WHOLENESS

*When we find the place of our own resurrection, we find
the truth of our own soul and purpose for which we were born.
This truth liberates us to live the unique and authentic life.*
                                            Karla Kincannon[57]

I had just received a message that indicated I would be landing in a Central American country I had never been to before—alone. I froze; my stomach ached, my breathing tightened, my thinking clouded. I was in a box with the walls closing in on me and I could not move. Suddenly I was back on the stretcher, not knowing where I was or what was happening, abandoned by my safe-keepers—alone in unknown territory and swirling in another world. There the Drama thoughts poured in: "I am just going to call and say I can't go." "I should have found out about this earlier. I always make assumptions and get myself in trouble." "They should have told me I was going to be alone." "You're a big girl now. You can do this", trying to puff myself up from the inside out so I looked like the Pillsbury Dough Boy—full of hot air! One pinprick would have easily deflated me.

I took in a deep breath, bent over while holding onto my stomach, and looked at my feet. As quickly as I had time traveled to three-stepping on the Drama Dance floor, I was back to earth and on solid ground. After doing the six-pointed star meditation, I asked myself: "What do I need?" I knew immediately: Safety. Helper? Truth. Action: Ask for what I need from person planning the trip. Student? I am. Teacher? Trip planner. Knowledge? I still live as if I am an abandoned child. Death? The belief that "I am always abandoned." Birth? I am adult who can stay with and keep myself safe. Living? Keep myself safe by providing for my safety needs. In this case, keeping myself safe involved contacting the trip planner and expressing my concerns. When I emailed the trip planner, her response was on target: "Do not worry, Bonnie. I will not abandon you!"

Early the next morning, I lay in bed with my one hand on my brow and one in the root chakra, just letting the healing energies come to me. As I did this I became aware, deep, deep within that "I am scared." I felt the flooding of

---

[57] Karla Kincannon p.213

the energies surround me as the presence of Compassion poured in. These healing energies seemed to get into even the tiniest specks of the scared me. That tiny child of old and this weathered adult of now joined hearts: scared <u>and</u> loved, frightened <u>and</u> accepted, fearful <u>and</u> present.

As I write these words, deep sobbing begins and I hold my heart, willing and able to be present to that long ago and still abandoned child. For healing does not mean she disappears — like some kind of magical zapping. Healing means that she gets to be a full member of the household that is Bonnie, with all the rights and privileges. She gets to have full status. She no longer has to live in the basement of the basement. She does not have to get it together, to puff herself up, or to pretend she is brave. She gets to have someone she can trust be present with her and hold her heart.

We have traveled full circle, from innocence as a natural mammal, through separation as a too excellent dancer of drama, through initiation, taking us through the three turns of the kaleidoscope, and returning again to wholeness. Along the way, self-love, truth, forgiveness, compassion, wisdom and higher purpose have been our constant companions.

By turning the kaleidoscope just slightly and adding a tiny sliver more of light, a complete picture emerges. In our hearts, our playful, capable, powerful, innocent, vulnerable, and needy selves are restored. Now we can live our natural mammal selves surrounded in the crystalline six-pointed star of truth, self-love, forgiveness, higher purpose, compassion and wisdom. We get to be restored in such a way that we can be wild and powerful **and** compassionate and forgiving; we can know ourselves as needy as well as immersed in truth and higher purpose, We can know ourselves and this miraculous universe as whole.

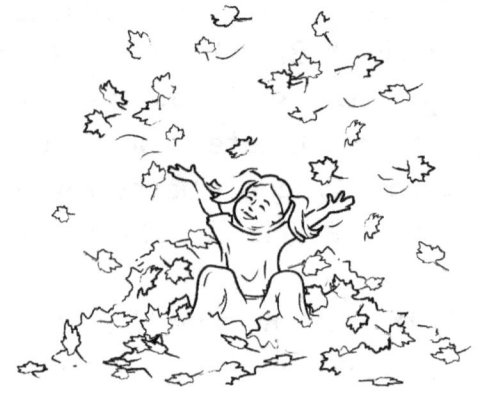

And so we have returned to where we began: full of delight. We reach our hands upward, tilt our heads to sky and let the leaves of love and peace and joy fall all over us.

Part VI: RESOURCES

Energetic Support System

Personal Stories of Healing the Victim Within

Quick! What's Your First Thought?

Complete Step-By-Step Overview

Bibliography

NOTES:

Energetic Support System

This section covers the hands-on energetic healing techniques and meditations, which provide the higher vibrations for the Healing-The-Victim-Within processes. Choose the energetic healings first, last and in between. When in doubt or stalled, choose and do an energetic healing technique or meditation.

The healing techniques include:

Amygdala Connection de-activates stuck reactive patterns to perceived life-threatening situations. It helps persons with post-traumatic stress syndrome, chronic patterns of fear, panic and anxiety by assisting in a shift out of fear-based energetic patterns. This shift opens energetic pathways for a new response of calm and compassion to previously perceived threatening situations. Pages 121-123.

Brain Connection helps the lower (action), middle (emoting) and upper (thinking) parts of the brain to work together and minimizes the domination of one part of the brain over the other two. Page 124.

Chakra Correspondence brings the support of the higher vibrational frequencies of the upper to the lower energy centers. This provides additional energetic support for information to be processed in a new way through the lower chakras. Page 125.

Quieting Hyper-Arousal of Fight-or-Flight calms or quiets the hyper-arousal of the fight or flight survival response. Page 126.

Shift-of-Consciousness Breathing easily and gently assists a change from being "asleep" in the Drama Dance to being "awake" in Three Turns of the Kaleidoscope. Page 127.

Tapping for Changing Habitual Hyper-arousal Reactions interrupts a habitual hyper-arousal or "kindling" and provides a healthier response to certain thoughts or situations. Page 128.

Three Gates and Three Cauldrons provides an energetic alignment of Physical Vitality, Heart's Desire, and Wisdom in order that a person might have the life energy to live her/his heart's desire or longing for the Beloved with Wisdom. Pages 129-131.

The healing meditations are:

Rosa Mystica Meditation invokes "protection through concentric circles of saints, healers, spiritual guides, and angels..." It may be used alone or in preparation for activities, such a completing the Three Turns or before participating in an activity, such as a family picnic, that triggers the Drama Dance in you. Page 132.

Six-Pointed Star: Healing Meditation is the first preparatory step in Healing-the-Victim-Within. In addition, this healing way may also be repeated as often as additional energetic support is needed. A powerful and transformational configuration, it is an energetic gateway for healing. Pages 30-31.

Amygdala Connection

Source: Marty Rather[58] and Bonnie Johnson, transcribers of this healing technique, received this spiritual guided information and named it the Amygdala Connection. The PBS Series – *The Secret Life of the Brain* – was a catalyst for Marty and Bonnie to seek guidance for a healing way for chronic anxiety and fear.

Purpose: De-activate stuck reactive patterns to perceived life-threatening situations. It helps persons with post-traumatic stress syndrome, chronic patterns of fear, panic and anxiety, by assisting them to a shift out of fear-based energetic patterns. This shift opens energetic pathways for a new response of calm and compassion to previously perceived threatening situations.

This particular healing sequence may provide long-lasting changes in one session.

Preparation:

- Prepare your mental understanding of the relevant anatomical structures by reviewing the drawing below.

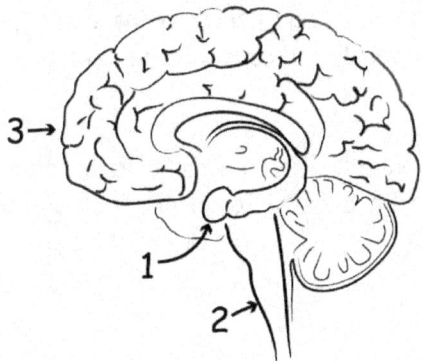
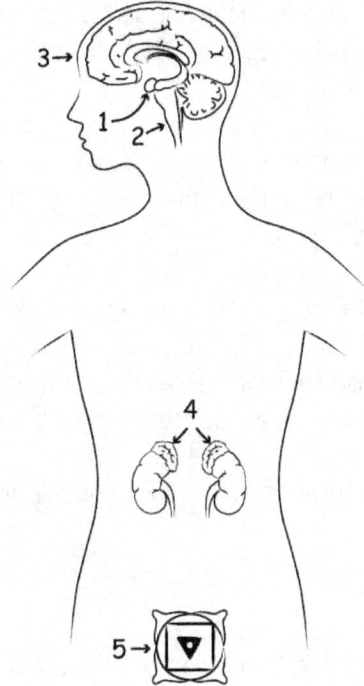

1. AMYGDALA
2. BRAIN STEM
3. PREFRONTAL CORTEX
4. ADRENALS
5. ROOT CHAKRA

- Identify the location of the amygdala, the brain stem and the pre-frontal cortex in the brain; the adrenal glands under the last ribs on the torso back; and the root energy center at the level of the tailbone at the base of spine. See descriptions of the purpose and function of these body parts in the background information.

---

[58] Above graphics designed by Marty Rather who is an energetic healer, artist and Vedic astrologist in Brentwood, Tennessee. She may be contacted by email: martyrather@comcast.net

Amygdala Connection (con't)

-Prepare yourself for giving and receiving healing by eliminating distractions. Quiet yourself. Ask yourself what you would like to receive in this healing. Release that request to the Highest Good for yourself and the whole universe. Then focus your attention on the healing process. You may also ask for the presence of Divine helpers.

<u>Process</u>:

1. Place the fingers of one hand so that tips of fingers point through back portion of top of head toward the Amygdala in center of brain. Make contact with and become aware of the energy of the Amygdala, by saying: "I am now contacting the Amygdala." Continue for one to five minutes to allow the healing energies to restore the energies of the Amygdala to a harmonious, balanced, soft golden radiance.

2. Keeping fingers on the Amygdala, place other hand on the brain stem (fingers at base of skull and pointing into and toward the brain). Hold this position until the Amygdala and brain stem are quiet and easily "communicating."

3. Keeping fingers on the Amygdala, place other hand on the prefrontal cerebral cortex (hand at front part of top of head and edge of brow). Hold this position until the Amygdala and cerebral cortex are quiet and easily "communicating."

4. Keeping fingers on the Amygdala move other hand from the prefrontal cerebral cortex to one adrenal gland. Hold this position until the Amygdala and adrenal are quiet and easily "communicating." Repeat with other adrenal gland.

5. Connect each adrenal with the root chakra.

6. Leave hand at root chakra and return fingers of other hand to the Amygdala. Hold this position until the Amygdala and root are quiet and easily "communicating."

7. Rest both hands on the heart. Sit quietly until ready to resume normal activities.

<u>NOTES:</u>

1. The Amygdala Connection may be repeated as needed. The energetic healing changes last from one session to next. Each subsequent session starts from the new energetic state, not from the same place as the first session.

2. This healing intervention increases the radiance of compassionate energy (even in previously or logically perceived life-threatening situations). It helps us move out of reacting from our first three chakras and into communicating with the love energy of the heart chakra.

In addition, a strong, higher vibrational base energy is infusing the earth planes. Many people have reacted to these new energies as if the energies were life threatening. The "Amygdala Connection" helps persons to receive these new foundational energies with their heart chakras open and filled with compassion.

© 2008 Three Turns of a Kaleidoscope by Bonnie Johnson - Permission granted to duplicate for personal and educational purposes.

Amygdala Connection (con't)

Background Information: The Amygdala is part of the limbic system, which is the emotional center or middle brain. This brain tissue is part of the first alert response to danger. When danger is perceived, before the person has any conscious awareness of danger, the Amygdala has detected and alerted the brain stem to react (fight or flee). The classic example, as featured in the PBS Brain series, is: you are walking down a path when you stop in mid-step. Your right leg bent at knee and held high over a long curving thing on the path. As you take a deep relaxing breath in, you laugh lightly and say: "Oh, it's just a stick." If the stick had been a snake, your Amygdala would have done its job in preventing you from walking right into the snake's danger zone.

The Brain Stem, located at the base of the brain, is the instinctual, automatic lower brain. We live as long as this part of the brain is functioning. It controls heart beating and respiratory function as well as automatic muscular reactions. The Brain Stem sends the message to your leg to stop mid-step.

The Pre-Frontal Cortex is the newest, evolutionary and development wise, kid on the brain block. Often called the upper or higher brain, it processes high intellectual and complex discernment processes. The Amygdala only needed a vague impression of the shape of the stick to alert the Brain Stem. The Pre-Frontal Cortex perceives multiple gradations of information to discern that the shape was not a dangerous snake but instead a harmless stick.

The Adrenal Glands produce the biochemical adrenaline, also known as the fight-or-flight hormone. When the Brain Stem receives the message of danger from the Amygdala, it sends a message to the Adrenals to produce and send adrenaline to the body, particularly the muscles, so that the physical body can fight or flee. It takes an increased heart rate, deeper breathing, increased blood sugar and muscle power to fight or flee. The Adrenals do their part to make that happen.

The Root Chakra or energy center, connects us, grounds and roots us to the energies of the planet earth. The earth has a powerful electro-magnetic field that feeds and nourishes us continuously. The energies that we experiences as strength, protection, plugged-in, safety, security, aliveness, vitality, and a sure trust in our own abilities and in our environment are processed by the root chakra. It encodes messages that help us to detect and avoid danger. In the human energy model, the root chakra detects the possible danger first before the physical body. It is the job of the root chakra to ensure that the physical body continues to be alive.

Brain Connection

Purpose:

To help the lower (action), middle (emoting) and upper (thinking) parts of the brain to work together and minimize the domination of one part of the brain over the other two

Preparation:

1. Prepare your mental understanding of the relevant anatomical and energetic structures by reviewing the drawing below. Identify the location of the upper, middle and lower brains as well as the root, sacral, solar plexus, heart, throat, brow and crown chakras.

2. Prepare yourself for giving and receiving healing by eliminating distractions. Quiet yourself. Ask yourself what you would like to receive in this healing. Release that request to the Highest Good for yourself and the whole universe. Then focus your attention on the healing process. You may also ask for the presence of Divine helpers.

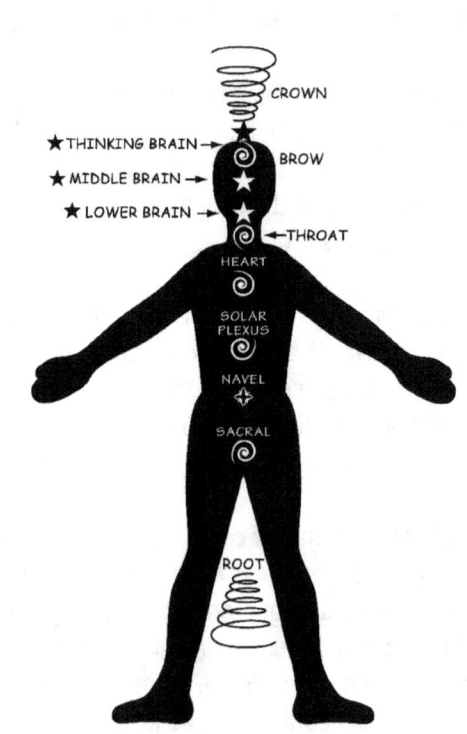

Process:

1. Place the fingers of your left hand in the groove in the middle of the base of skull. Connect with the lower brain (the action brain). When the connection is made, place your right hand into the root chakra. Connect the lower brain and root chakra. Then, move your right hand to the throat chakra. Connect the lower brain and throat chakra. Move your right hand to the heart chakra. Connect the lower brain and heart chakra.

2. Place the fingers of your left hand on the back of the head and connect with the middle brain (limbic system, the emotional brain). Then place your right hand into the sacral chakra. Connect with the middle brain with the sacral chakra. Move your right hand to the brow chakra. Connect with the middle brain with the brow chakra. Move your right hand to the heart chakra. Connect with the middle brain with the heart chakra.

3. Place your left hand on the top of the head and connect with cerebral cortex (thinking brain). Then place your right hand into the solar plexus. Connect the cerebral cortex with the solar plexus. Move your right hand to the crown chakra (or let the left hand do "double duty"). Connect the cerebral cortex with the crown chakra. Move your right hand to the heart chakra. Connect the cerebral cortex with the heart chakra.

4. Place both hands in the heart chakra. Rest quietly until ready to resume normal activities.

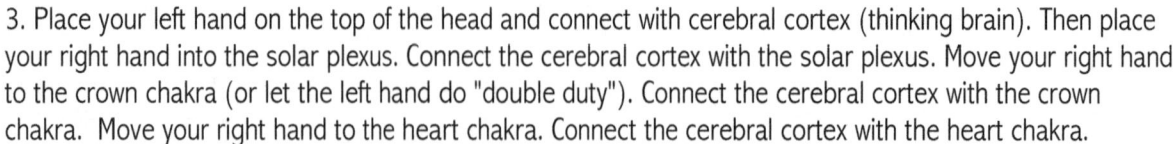

© 2008 Three Turns of a Kaleidoscope by Bonnie Johnson – Permission granted to duplicate for personal and educational purposes.

Chakra Correspondence

Purpose:
To bring the higher vibrational frequencies of the upper to the lower energy centers. This provides additional energetic support for information to be processed in a new way through the lower chakras for Healing-The-Victim-Within.

Preparation:

Prepare yourself for giving and receiving healing by eliminating distractions. Quiet yourself. Ask yourself what you would like to receive in this healing. Release that request to the Highest Good for yourself and the whole universe. Then focus your attention on the healing process. You may also ask for the presence of Divine helpers.

Process:

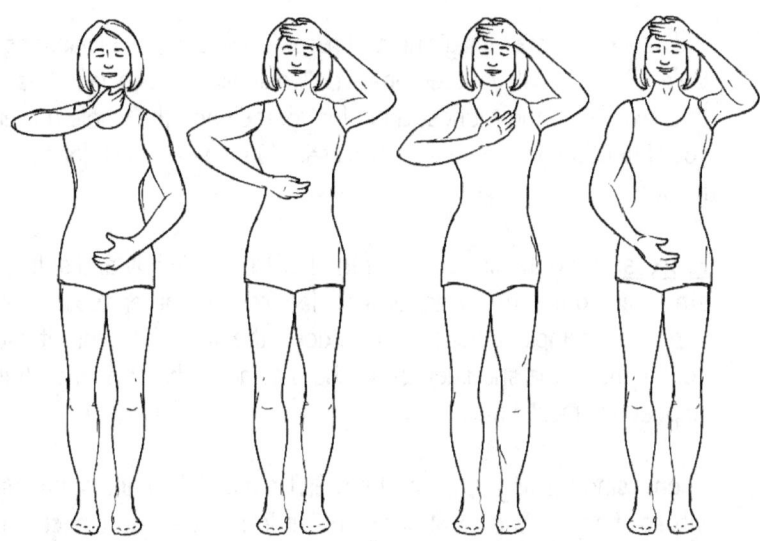

Place one hand in either the root, sacral, solar plexus or heart chakra.

Place the other hand in the throat chakra. Ask or have the intention for the energies and qualities of truth, forgiveness or self-love to infuse the lower chakra where the other hand is positioned. This will help in the healing process for each of the healing triangles.

OR

Place the other hand in the brow chakra. Ask or have the intention for the energies and qualities of wisdom, compassion or higher purpose to infuse the lower chakra where the other hand is positioned. This will help in the healing process for each of the healing triangles.

OR

Place the other hand in the crown chakra. Ask or have the intention for the energies and qualities of wisdom, compassion, higher purpose, truth, forgiveness and self-love to infuse the lower chakra where the other hand is positioned. This will help in the healing process for each of the healing triangles. This position is especially helpful at the heart level of the Death-Birth-Life triangle.

Quieting Hyper-Arousal of Fight-or-Flight

Source: *Energy Medicine* by Donna Eden

Purpose: to calm or quiet the hyper-arousal of the fight or flight survival response

Preparation:

1. Look at drawing below. Note the dotted line from the outer aspect of the eye, across the temple, behind the ear, down the side of the throat, along the collarbone to the shoulder, down the outside of the arm, and off the fourth finger. This represents the Triple Warmer meridian as described in Chinese Traditional Medicine. Its function in the human body corresponds to the fight-or-flight response described in conventional western medicine.

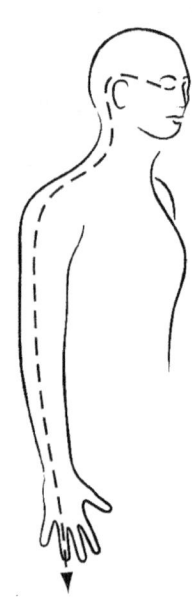

2. Prepare yourself for giving and receiving healing by eliminating distractions. Quiet yourself. Ask yourself what you would like to receive in this healing. Release that request to the Highest Good for yourself and the whole universe. Then focus your attention on the healing process. You may also ask for the presence of Divine helpers.

Process: Using the finger tips of the LEFT hand, lightly and softly, barely touching, stroke along the triple warmer meridian from the outer aspect of the RIGHT eye, across the temple, behind the ear, down the side of the throat, along the collarbone to the shoulder, down the outside of the arm, and off the fourth finger. Repeat two more times.

Then, using the finger tips of the RIGHT hand, lightly and softly, barely touching, stroke along the triple warmer meridian from the outer aspect of the LEFT eye, across the temple, behind the ear, down the side of the throat, along the collarbone to the shoulder, down the outside of the arm, and off the fourth finger. Repeat two more times.

Place both hands in the heart chakra. Rest quietly until ready to resume normal activities.

Shift-of-Consciousness Breathing

<u>Purpose</u>: to create a shift in consciousness to move a person out of the Drama Dance and into Three Turns of the Kaleidoscope: Healing The Victim Within.

<u>Process</u>:

Take a breather:
Look down at your feet.
Bend over, so your head and arms hang down loosely and come closer to your feet.
Breathe as you notice the air come in and out through your nose and mouth.

<u>Background</u>:

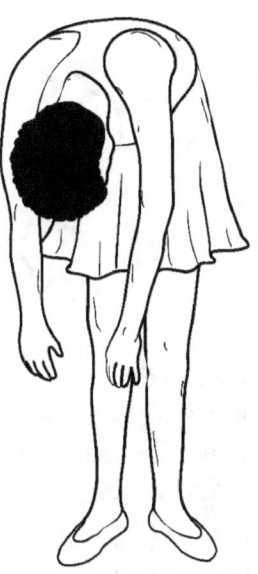

When we take a breather, literally stop and breathe in and out, and look down at our feet, we have a chance to ask and discover what all the mad dancing is about. For all you non-dancers or non-runners out there, go to a dance place or runners' route and watch people as they dance or run. Notice that dancers or runners, when they pause to "catch their breath," all breathe deeply and lower their heads and eyes to their feet. They sometimes bend way over with their heads coming quite close to their feet. These movements of the physical body bring dancers and runners back to earth, grounding them, and helping them to refill their energetic stores used in the dancing or running. This helps them to restore literal balance, so they can continue to dance or run in rhythm.

Tapping for Changing Habitual Hyper-arousal Reactions

Source: *Energy Medicine* by Donna Eden

Purpose: To change habitual hyper-arousal or kindling to certain thoughts or situations

Preparation:

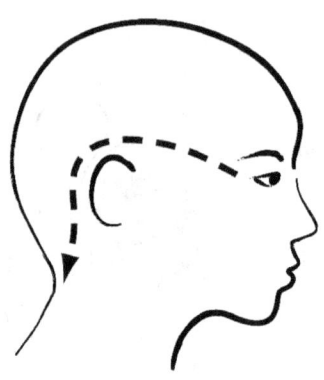

1. Look at the drawing and note the meridian represented as a dotted line from the outer aspect of the eye, across the temple, behind the ear, and to the base of skull. This is the beginning portion of the Triple Warmer meridian as described in Chinese Traditional Medicine. The function of this meridian corresponds to the fight-or-flight response described in conventional western medicine.

2. Choose a thought, behavior or situation that usually elicits anxiousness, worry, obsessive thinking or behaviors, panicky feelings or fear.

3. Then, decide how you would like to respond. Write this new way as a short sentence. Then rewrite the sentence in a negative form that still communicates the same message. For example: "I am calm and confident when attending parties." The rewrite in negative form: "I am no longer nervous and unsure when attending parties."

4. Prepare yourself for giving and receiving healing by eliminating distractions. Quiet yourself. Ask yourself what you would like to receive in this healing. Release that request to the Highest Good for yourself and the whole universe. Then focus your attention on the healing process. You may also ask for the presence of Divine helpers.

Process:

Place the fingers of the RIGHT hand at the RIGHT temple. Tap gently along the meridian from temple, behind the ear, down the side of the throat, to base of skull while saying positive message. For example, I would tap and say: "I am calm and confident when attending parties." Let your words and tappings correspond in a rhythmic pattern. Repeat words and tappings for a total of FIVE times.

Place the fingers of the LEFT hand at the LEFT temple. Tap gently along the meridian from temple, behind the ear, down the side of the throat, to base of skull while saying negatively phrased message. For example, I would tap and say: "I am no longer nervous and unsure when attending parties." Let your words and tappings correspond in a rhythmic pattern. Repeat words and tappings for a total of FIVE times.

Place both hands in the heart chakra. Rest quietly until ready to resume normal activities.

You may do the tappings as many times in one day as desired and for as many days until you no longer feel the need. Often, you will just forget to do the tapping. This forgetting will naturally indicate a completion. Weeks, months or even years later, if an additional boost is needed, the whole process may be repeated.

Three Gates and Three Cauldrons

Purpose:

To align Physical Vitality, Heart's Desire, and Wisdom in order that a person might have the life energy to live the heart's desire or longing for the Beloved with Wisdom

Preparation:

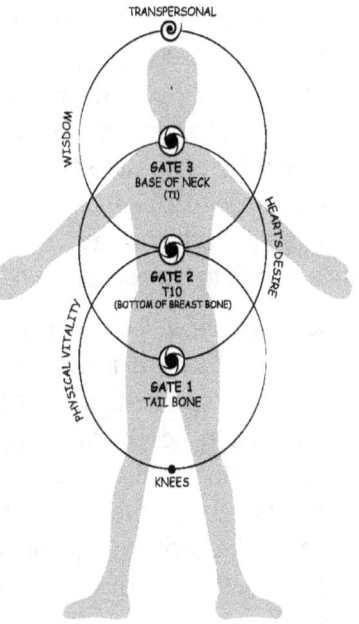

1. View drawing for the positions of three energetic gates in relation to the physical spine. Notice also the placement of the three energetic circles or "cauldrons".

2. Prepare yourself for giving and receiving healing by eliminating distractions. Quiet yourself. Ask yourself what you would like to receive in this healing. Release that request to the Highest Good for yourself and the whole universe. Then focus your attention on the healing process. You may also ask for the presence of Divine helpers.

Process:

The first energetic gate is located at the tailbone at the base of the physical spine. This gate opens and closes similar to purse strings or the iris of an eye. It controls the inflow of energy that vitalizes the physical body.

1. Place one hand over your lower spine (the tailbone) while you visualize this energetic gate. This might look like a circular iris or purse strings that close and open. This expanding and constricting of the gate controls the flow of energy through the gate. Invite Healing Energy to flow into this energetic gate so the qualities of ease and flexibility may be incorporated into the energetic structure of the gate. When you have a sense of the gate being able to open and close easily, continue to allow the Healing energy to activate the physical vitality energies. You may sense this activation as a strong vibration. Wait for the strong vibration to become smooth before moving to next step.

The second gate is located at the level of tenth thoracic vertebrae, directly behind the bottom of the sternum or chest bone. This gate opens and closes similar to the iris of an eye or purse strings. It controls the inflow of energy that vitalizes the heart's desire, the deep longing for the Beloved or one's soul purpose.

2. Move the hand from the tailbone area to area of the tenth thoracic vertebrae. Visualize this energetic gate. This might look like a circular iris or purse strings that constrict and expand. This expanding and constricting of the gate controls the flow of energy through the gate. Invite Healing Energy to flow into this energetic gate so that the qualities of ease and flexibility may be incorporated into the energetic structure of this gate. When you have a sense of the gate being able to open and close easily, continue to allow the Healing Energy to activate the energies that support and nourish the heart's desire. You may sense this activation as warm and sweet infusion. Wait for energies to be smooth and even before moving to the next step.

© 2008 Three Turns of a Kaleidoscope by Bonnie Johnson – Permission granted to duplicate for personal and educational purposes.

Three Gates and Three Cauldrons (con't)

The third gate is located at the juncture of the last cervical and first thoracic vertebrae. Slide your fingers down the spine from the base of the skull until the fingers encounter the first bumpy vertebrae. This is the location of the third gate. This gate also opens and closes similar to the iris or purse strings. It controls the in flow of energy that enhances or augments Wisdom.

3. Move the hand to rest under the third gate at the juncture of the last cervical and first thoracic vertebrae or big bump. Visualize this energetic gate. This might look like a circular iris or purse strings that constrict and expand. This expanding and constricting of the gate controls the flow of energy through the gate. Invite Healing Energy to flow into this energetic gate so that the qualities of ease and flexibility may be incorporated into the energetic structure of this gate. When you have a sense of the gate being able to open and close easily, continue to allow the Healing Energy to activate the energies that support and nourish Wisdom. You may sense this activation as a smooth circular or spiral movement. Wait for energies to be smooth and even before moving to the next step.

4. Place one hand at the level of and between your knees, with palm facing toward the head; place the other hand at level of second gate at the base of the chest bone, with palm facing toward the feet. The first gate at the base of the spine is the center of this circle. Imagine that your palms are resting on a large circle, such as a bubble, egg, bowl or cauldron, as the healing energies known as life force, prana or chi fills this circle. You may wish to intentionally breathe in deeply, and then as you breathe out, imagine the Divine Breath filling this cauldron. Next, move your hands from the top and bottom of the cauldron to the sides of the cauldron and then to the back and front of the cauldron. Become aware of the size of this energy bubble. Notice that it is filled with the nourishing energies that fortify your physical vitality.

5. Place one hand at level of first gate at the base of the spine, with palm facing toward the head; place the other hand at level of third gate right below your chin, with palm facing toward the feet. The second gate at the base of the chest bone is the center of this circle. Imagine that your palms are resting on a large circle, such as a bubble, egg, bowl or cauldron, as the healing energies known as life force, prana or chi fills this circle. You may wish to intentionally breathe deeply in, and then as you breathe out, imagine the Divine Breath filling this cauldron. Next, move your hands from the top and bottom of the cauldron to the sides of the cauldron and then to the back and front of the cauldron. Become aware of the size of this energy bubble. Notice that it is filled with the nourishing energies that fortify your heart's desire, soul purpose or longing for the Beloved.

6. Place one hand at level of second gate at the base of the chest bone, with palm facing toward the head; place the other hand at level of transpersonal point 18 inches above the top of your head, with palm facing toward the feet. The third gate at the "big bump" is the center of this circle. Imagine that your palms are resting on a large circle, such as a bubble, egg, bowl or cauldron, as the healing energies known as life force, prana or chi fills this circle. You may wish to intentionally breathe deeply in, and then as you breathe out, imagine the Divine Breath filling this cauldron. Next, move your hands from the top and bottom of the cauldron to the sides of the cauldron and then to the back and front of the cauldron. Become aware of the size of this energy bubble. Notice that it is filled with the nourishing energies that fortify Wisdom.

© 2008 Three Turns of a Kaleidoscope by Bonnie Johnson – Permission granted to duplicate for personal and educational purposes.

Three Gates and Three Cauldrons (con't)

7. Place both hands in the heart chakra. Be aware of the energetic alignment along your spine of vitality, heart's desire and wisdom, and of the three nourishing energetic cauldrons.

When ready, you may resume normal activities.

<u>Source and Background Information</u>: This healing intervention came to me in Guidance when I was providing a healing for a client in early 2000.

In my training as an energetic healer, I had been introduced to different teachings that have similarities. In the early nineties Mia Beale, a healer in Maine taught me a technique she called the "egg" which she had learned from healer par excellence Roslyn Bruyere. My memory of this teaching was of three energetic eggs that provide long-lasting nourishment for the person's continued healing. In my Tai Ji classes, I learned "Swimming Dragon" which includes a movement of the hands that "traces" three circles twice!

Deep gratitude goes to Celtic shaman and author Frank MacEowen, who poetically describes and names these three circles in *The Mist-Filled Path*. From him I have borrowed the term cauldron as homage to my rich Celtic heritage as well as the transformational images that cauldron provokes. He also uses the words life force, calling, and wisdom for the three cauldrons, providing energetic corroboration for the guided information I had received.

The energetic gates, especially the T10 gate, revealed themselves in individual healings. I first became aware of T10 gate after reading about de-energizing elementals (thought forms) in *Fire In The Heart* by Kyriacos C. Markides. Since the book gave no directions on how to de-energize a thought form, I went into a deep meditative state and asked for directions. The information I received included directions for working with the T10 gate. In Traditional Chinese teachings of the Microcosmic Orbit Flow, particularly the work of Mantak Chia, I learned of energetic gates or openings that were important to free flowing energy along the central meridian pathway.

From Mary Magdalena came the information of the three gates and cauldrons aligned and filled bringing together the energies of the divine masculine (first gate and circle) and the divine feminine (third gate and circle) connected through the second gate and circle which are the energies of the heart's longing.

Our whole beings long for, search all our lives, and weep with joy when we know ourselves as this wholeness, this holiness.

Rosa Mystica Meditation

A litany is one of the oldest forms of liturgical prayer, sung in a series of repeated invocations or commemorations.... The ancient Irish word that translates as litany means "shield".... The practice of invoking protection from concentric circles of saints and angels Therese Schroeder-Sheker[59]

This healing meditation was inspired by and adapted from a description of the litany of the Rosa Mystica by Therese Schroeder-Sheker. This meditation may be used alone or in preparation for activities, such as completing the Three Turns of the Kaleidoscope or before participating in an activity, for example a family picnic, that triggers the Drama Dance in you.

Prepare yourself for meditation by creating a space with as few distractions as possible. Sit or lie in a way that is physically comfortable for you. Let your attention move to your mid-chest. Quietly, observe yourself, breathing in and breathing out. No need to change your breathing; just let your attention be with your breathing for a few minutes.

Begin by imagining yourself as the center of a beautiful rosebud.

The first layer of rose petals is your first layer of protection and help. Name them, calling them forth to be with you. This might be your grandmother or grandfather or a dear and wise elder in your life, one who may have passed on to the other worlds.

The second layer of rose petals is your second layer of protection and help. Name them, calling them forth to be with you. These may be significant healing beings who have lived on this earth: Mother Theresa, Princess Diane, Hildegard von Bingden...

The third layer of rose petals is your third layer of protection and help. Name them, calling them forth to be with you. These may be avatars or great spiritual beings: Mother Mary, Mary Magdalena, Brigid...

The fourth layer of rose petals is your fourth layer of protection and help. Name them, calling them forth to be with you. These are angelic beings and goddesses: Isis, Kwan Yin...

The fifth layer of rose petals is your fifth layer of protection and help. Call them forth to be with you, aware that this layer is the UNnameable, the Unmanifested: Shekinah, Sophia, Shakti...

Rest in this awareness.

---

[59] http://www.cduniverse.com/search/xx/music/pid/1008570/a/Rosa+Mystica.htm

Personal Stories
Of
Healing the Victim Within

1. An Old Story: Yamina

2. Dramatic Food: Rene

3. A Love Story: Melodie

© 2008 Three Turns of a Kaleidoscope by Bonnie Johnson – Permission granted to duplicate for personal and educational purposes.

NOTES:

An Old Story: Yamina

Yamina is a fifty-five year-old woman with a quick wit, sensitive nature, kind heart and artistic gifts. She is a fiber artist (spinning and dyeing the wool she knits into colorful shawls, socks, scarves), a Vedic astrologer, businesswoman, writer and healer. Her story begins with her childhood and vividly conveys the long-lasting effects of socialization and the ensuing Drama. The healing process she describes began and occurred mostly in a one-day workshop titled "Healing The Inner Victim".

Yamina's father had polio as a child that left him disabled; this disease contributed to his Persecution of both Yamina and her mother. In Yamina's mind, he was the Persecutor, she and her mother were the innocent Victims. Now as she looks back, she can clearly see how they all exchanged positions on the Drama Triangle, each of them taking turns playing the Victim, Persecutor and Rescuer with each other. Yamina describes it as "chasing each other around the triangle." Let's listen in as Yamina tells her story of healing the Victim within:

"My Dad's Persecution was mostly psychological in nature. Out of his human love for me, he wanted to and tried to give me useful skills for life. Due to his polio-caused disability, his perception of life was often distorted. A mild example is his teaching me to drive a car using only one hand. This worked well for him because his right hand was non-functional but not for me. This is just one of many such seemingly innocent yet hurtful examples.

"However, the most distorted programming came in the phrase he used every time I would approach him with a problem. 'Yamina,' Dad would say, 'you don't have polio. You don't have any problems.' I must have heard this a thousand times while growing up." When Yamina tried to defend herself — often with great skill — the drama took another switch: "Mom would encourage me to 'listen to your father,' adding a layer of drama intensity which Rescued him and Persecuted me." At this point, Yamina would switch to Rescuer by waiting on her father. She would say: "Poor Dad, he has polio. I need to take care of him." Or, she would Rescue herself by going off by herself to play. She would advise herself: "No one is going to look out for you but yourself. You are all alone, so it is best to make the most of it." Then, she spent hours by herself. As she played, the Persecutor would raise its head to shame her with these words: "Yamina, you are so pitiful. Even your parents don't want to play with you."

Yamina was in her forties when she began to wonder: "Why do I have so many problems? I don't have polio!" She noted: "Not having polio was not much of a problem-solving skill. With many problems and few problem-solving skills I needed help! That's when I started taking self-help and inner-study workshops. The anger inside me was just starting to come out. The more I learned, the angrier I exclaimed 'poor me.' Living life as not-a-cripple is undermining in itself. It is just not the same as living a healthy and successful life. In experiencing life, through the lens of not-a-cripple, I encountered self-limiting and painful thoughts that led to anger, unhappiness and a lot of confusion. It is true that I was not-a-cripple, but it is not the whole truth. It is a debilitating truth."

"Finally, in the 'Healing the Inner Victim' workshop, I was able to see the depths and futility of this programming, and a way to climb out of it. "

Here is the healing the Victim within process that Yamina used to address her Drama:

1. Drama Triangle

Yamina described and identified her Drama and the roles she played: "I had to define the wound and admit to playing all three parts in the Drama triangle. It was easier to see Mom and Dad playing all three parts, but eventually I could see my own part more clearly."

RESCUER

"It's okay, Yamina. You can go play by yourself. No one will bother you then."

PERSECUTOR

"Yamina, you don't have polio. You don't have any problems."

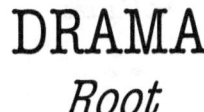

DRAMA
Root

VICTIM

"Poor little me."

2. Need-Help-Action Triangle

"I realized that I had already taken the step of asking for help from people I trusted by taking workshops to learn problem-solving skills, although my resentment against my father initially increased." Note: This increase in anger is a reflection of moving from powerless to powerful.

<u>HELP</u>

"Truth."

<u>ACTION</u>

"Learn problem-solving skills."

EMOTIONS
Sacral

<u>NEED</u>

"Trust."

3. Student-Teacher-Knowledge Triangle

"This is where I discovered how I had gotten confused. I finally saw the process of indoctrination I had gone through (instead of the random anger I had been feeling). Here Dad was the teacher and I was the student and the knowledge was distorted. But immediately I started seeing that not all of the knowledge was distorted. He had lots of good qualities as well. I started seeing the good and useful and funny things he had also taught me. The anger was surprisingly starting to subside. I can still go back to this triangle to get more information both helpful and distorted to work on clearing out."

KNOWLEDGE

"My Dad taught me both useful as well as useless information."

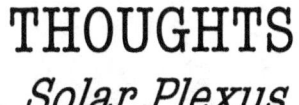

THOUGHTS
Solar Plexus

STUDENT

"I am."

TEACHER

"My Dad."

4. Death-Birth-Life Triangle

In exploring this healing triangle, Yamina answered the questions this way:

What needs to die? What false idea or belief is ready to be de-structed? "When Dad dies, I will be free of all his useless influence."

What new can be created out of that which has been de-structed? I can always remember Dad's good influence."

What can now be lived out of this new creation? "Discovering a new definition of Unconditional Love and Self-acceptance."

LIFE

"Discovering a new definition of Unconditional Love and Self-acceptance."

AWARENESS
Heart

BIRTH

"I can always remember Dad's good influence."

DEATH

"When Dad dies, I will be free of all his influence."

Yamina continues: "This information was powerfully overwhelming for me. To let go of my anger and move into unconditional love and self-acceptance all in one day was thoroughly exhausting. In truth, it was not until today (approximately one year later) that I completed the six-pointed star by putting the two "Qualities" triangles together with my own definitions for the words signifying each angle. Here is what I have discovered:

Wholeness:

1. I accept the <u>Truth</u> of these situations.
2. I can <u>forgive</u> others and myself for being "dramatic" imperfect humans.
3. I have learned to love myself (<u>Self Love</u>) as well as others unconditionally.
4. Freedom from attachment to drama allows <u>Wisdom</u> to flow into my life.
5. My heart and mind now expand with <u>Compassion</u> for all souls including my own.
6. The <u>Higher Purpose</u> of my life is revealed and embraced."

Rene's Story: Food and the Drama Dance

Rene is a sixty-four year old woman with a vibrant zest for living fully. She expresses an awareness of and a gratitude for all the blessings in her life. On this particular day, she has decided to focus on an experience she had the evening before.

She had a full day of nourishing herself with healthy and balanced foods and activities: walking on a glistening white beach along the Gulf of Mexico, doing Tai Ji and Yoga and quieting meditation, being with and sharing with a special friend, as well as reading a stimulating and reflective book. After a delicious snack, she and her friend parted ways for the night.

Rene noticed herself seeking food to eat. She was well aware that she was not physically hungry. Soon she found herself snacking on almonds. She began to question herself. "What is this feeling I am experiencing that starts me looking for food?" Then, she said to herself: "Well, you know you are a recovering food addict[60]. You just can't help yourself. You're just not capable of resisting food." Then she began to barrage herself with: "But why? What is wrong with me that I keep doing this?" Then she switched: "It's okay. You're doing the best you can."

Bonnie: Rene, let's start with something in your life that is bothering you or presenting itself as a problem. Something you would like to heal or get some help for. What would you like to focus on right now?

Rene: Heal the pattern of eating rather than experiencing the feelings that trigger the desire to eat when I am not hungry.

Bonnie: Tell me more about this pattern.

Rene: I want to be able to identify or recognize the feeling before eating. Last night, I had a great day. At the end of the day, I was alone, not hungry, felt full. I had just eaten my snack food. I got out and ate more snack food, while recognizing all the reasons not to eat it.

---

60 Food addiction is "the compulsive pursuit of a mood change by engaging repeatedly in episodes of binge eating despite adverse consequences" as defined by Kay Sheppard, p.3.

Bonnie: Let's look at this from the perspective of the Drama Dance. It is a way that we relate to ourselves and to others, [people, animals, objects, groups, institutions, gods, angels, and environment: sun, earth, water, rain] that keeps us in unhealthy self-perpetuating triangular pattern. Remember, there are three positions: Victim, Rescuer and Persecutor. These three positions or roles are ones we assume and switch rapidly from one to the other.

First, let's identify you in the Victim position.

Rene: "I can't control myself. I can't help it. I'm not capable. I'm no good."

Bonnie: Now, let's identify you in the Rescuer position.

Rene: "It's okay. You have an addiction and this just happens. You can do better tomorrow."

Bonnie: Now, let's identify you in the Persecutor position.

Rene: "You (speaking to herself) know how to do this – just do it! (with strong vocal emphasis). "Why do you keep doing this? You know better. You've been on this recovering food addict plan for years and know how it works, so just do it. You are a bad person."

Bonnie: Let's review. When you ate off the food plan last night, you were unaware of a feeling before you started eating extra food. You said: "I am powerless and no good." Then you patted yourself on the head (metaphorically) and said, "It's okay. You can do better tomorrow." Then you berated yourself and called yourself a bad person. Is that right?

Rene: Nods head up and down.

Bonnie: Let's get some energetic help. I am going to trace the six-pointed star in your energy system. Then I will show you how to do this meditation on yourself. (See pages 30-31 for diagram and description of the six-pointed star meditation.)

Now, let's look at the first healing triangle. The first healing triangle is need, help, and action. It is associated with ordinary emotions. It is the first step in restoring the healthy child as a healthy adult. It is the first step in healing this particular drama in your life.

Let's start with the need. When you were in the midst of the drama triangle, telling yourself, "I am powerless, no good," you patted yourself on the head (metaphorically) and said, "It's okay. You can do better tomorrow." Then you berated yourself and called yourself a bad person. What was the need right then? Remember the need is always related to trust, security, safety, survival or vitality. In this situation, what is the need? Let the first thing that comes to your mind be the answer.

Rene: Trust.

Bonnie: Okay, trust is the need. Let's look at the help. Remember the six-pointed star is made up of six qualities or qualities: truth, self-love, forgiveness, compassion, wisdom and higher purpose (See diagrams and descriptions on pages 103-114). Choose one of these qualities to help heal this particular drama. Again, let the first thing that comes to your mind be the answer.

Rene: Wisdom.

Bonnie: Knowing now that **trust** is the **need**, and **wisdom** is the **help**, what's the **action** for you? Again, let the first thing that comes to your mind be the answer.

Rene: (Hems and Haws for a minute) Meditate.

Bonnie: (Summarizing) In this drama situation, you had a good day, everything seemed fine, then you wanted to eat more. You identified that the need is related to trust, the quality for helping you is wisdom and the action is to meditate.

The second healing triangle is oriented toward conceptual thinking. The three positions are: student, teacher and knowledge. In this drama situation of good day, wanting to and eating more, who is the student, who is the teacher and what is the knowledge acquired? Let's start with who is the student?

Rene: I am the student. This seems obvious. Could it be someone else?

Bonnie: Yes, but most of the time it is the person seeking healing. Who is the teacher? Could be a person, aspect of self, an event, or situation... First thing that comes to mind.

Rene: Food is the teacher. (Sounds surprised and thoughtful).

Bonnie: You are the student; the food is the teacher. What are you learning from the food?

Rene: Food is not the answer.

Bonnie: Now, for the last healing triangle. This triangle is made up of death, birth and life. In order for this drama pattern to heal, something must be destructed, then something can be born or created, then that new creation can be lived. So imagine this something that needs to be destructed is made out of Lego blocks. You can destruct it as easily as taking the blocks apart.

What needs to be destructed? What needs to die?

Rene: The mistaken idea that food is the answer.

Bonnie: Okay, the idea "Food is the answer" is taken apart and dies. What is created? What is birthed out of the Lego blocks?

Rene: Identifying that feeling before I start eating too much.

Bonnie: No, that's where we started, this is something new. What is newly created?

Rene: (pausing)

Bonnie: First thought??

Rene: I don't know

Bonnie: You do not know. This new is the unknown or maybe the Unknown; a willingness to enter into the unknown/Unknown and just be there. This would be the third aspect: living this new creation. Are you willing? Remember, as you live in the unknown, you continue to have the quality of wisdom. You also have the other five qualities available: self-love, forgiveness, truth, compassion and higher purpose.

Rene: Yes, I'm willing.

Bonnie: Each day, trace the six-pointed star as I taught you. Let's review it again. You may do this as many times in a day as you desire or need.

Again, let's review: With the help of wisdom, you may meet the need of trusting through the action of meditating. You have learned that food is not the answer and willingly destructed this false idea of "Food is the answer." You recognize that food has been teaching this to you all along. What has been created out of this false belief is an awareness of the unknown. You are willing to live in the space of the unknown/Unknown.

Rene's Story: Food and the Drama Dance   147

Below are the completed triangles in diagram format:

1. Drama Triangle

RESCUER

*"It's okay. You have an addiction
and this just happens.
You can do better tomorrow."*

PERSECUTOR

*"You know how to do this –
just do it (with strong vocal emphasis)
You are a bad person!"*

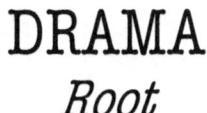

DRAMA
Root

VICTIM

*"I can't control myself.
I can't help it.
I'm not capable.
I'm no good."*

2. Need-Help-Action Triangle

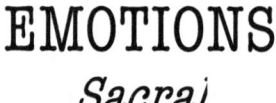

3. Student-Teacher-Knowledge Triangle

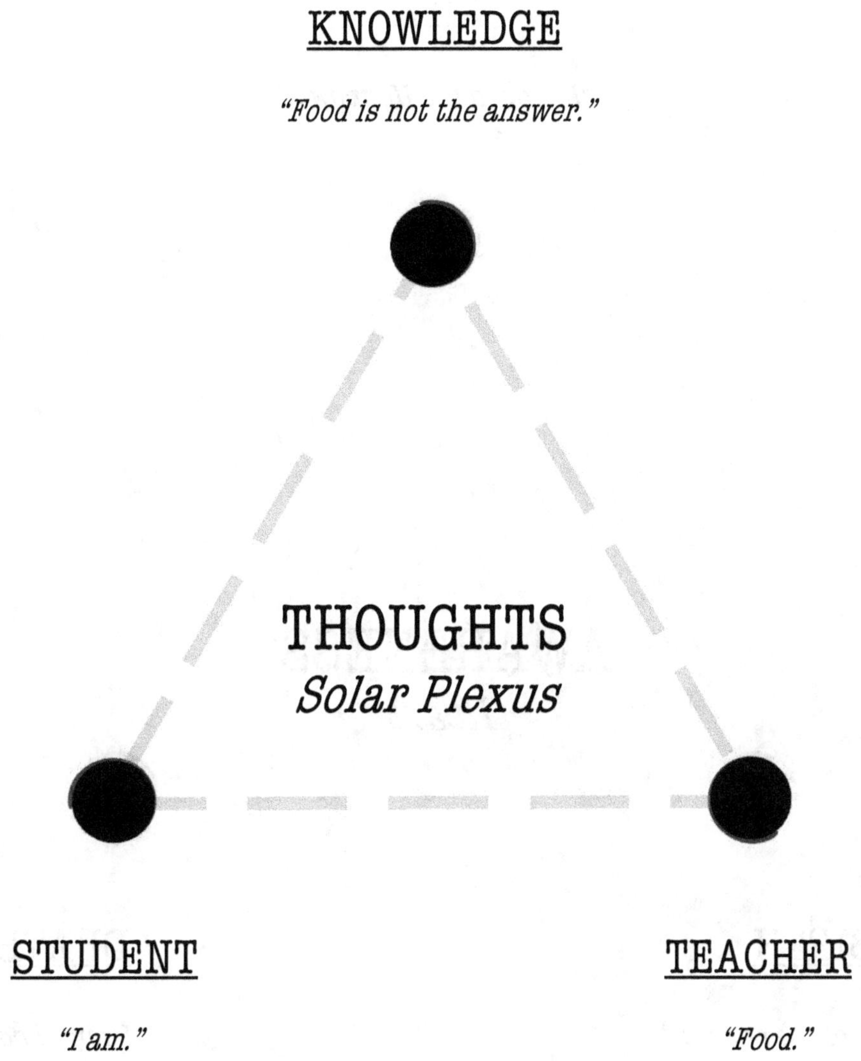

KNOWLEDGE

"Food is not the answer."

THOUGHTS
Solar Plexus

STUDENT

"I am."

TEACHER

"Food."

4. Death-Birth-Life Triangle

LIFE

"Living in the Unknown."

●

AWARENESS
Heart

● ●

BIRTH   # DEATH

"Food is not the answer."   *"I don't know."*

Four weeks later, Rene relates: "I found that I didn't do the exercises you recommended and I didn't even remember the information I discovered or how to do the triangles. I really didn't do anything with it.

My food addiction got worse and I spent a week with increased binging on food (and thoughts of food). I was increasingly spending more and more of my energy on food and less on the things in my life that needed or wanted doing. I saw myself spiraling downward and knew I didn't want to go there and that I needed help and lots of help.

I called my sponsor, my energetic healer, and my psychiatrist. After I received the energetic healing, things shifted. Once I saw and talked with my sponsor I was once again back in recovery. I know I have to have the supportive help. I cannot do this by myself. One of my long-standing beliefs is: I have to do everything myself and if I just think about something long and hard enough, I will be able fix what is wrong."

Bonnie's assessment: Even though Rene did not consciously use the healing the Victim within process in the weeks following the above session, it was energetically working in her life. First, in her description of spiraling downward, she had an increased observation of herself. She stood further back, providing more distance between herself binging and her greater, stronger, healthier observing self. This ability to "step back" from ourselves creates a detachment from the Drama and an attachment to the newly created life.

Second, her commitment to her healthy self reveals itself in an increased commitment to an ongoing spiritual practice that under-girds her vibrancy, and assists her to be solid and integrated into herself. She has moved from her recovery of just following the food plan and doing the twelve steps[61] in order to be healthy, to choosing a full vibrant life for herself. Following the food plan and twelve steps is the means she is choosing to get her there. The emphasis has shifted from doing to being.

---

[61] The twelve-step recovery program for food addictions is described in Kay Sheppard's Food Addiction, The Body Knows and follows the twelve-step format of the Alcoholics Anonymous recovery program.

Third, as she relayed her binge eating and binge thinking, her voice was matter-of-fact without any trace of Victim, Rescuer, or Persecutor. This lack of beating herself up for binging was a significant change.

Rene's addendum: I now recognize the "I don't know" answer as giving up control. I felt like the 'I don't know' answer was a failure to figure things out and do things the 'right' way. After another year of 12-step recovery work and energetic healings, I realized, as I re-read this story, that it was very complete. I gave up control without knowing it at the conscious level (where I was still in the Drama Dance). My wise teachers, guides and helpers (both visible and invisible) did and do what I cannot do alone.

A Love Story: Melodie

This story is an example of a minor, low-intensity Drama. The surface emotions in a minor drama are even enough that observation and examination can occur without kindling. In Rene and Yamina's drama stories, the Drama is long lived and the drama plot and lines well rehearsed. In this story, the characters have no prior drama experience with each other. Indeed, they have extensive experience in a trusting and healthy way of relating. However, Melodie has a lifetime of experiences drama dancing with her self. Let's have a look at how this minor Drama leads the way to deep and significant healing.

The drama scene: Lisa is arriving by plane Friday at 5:00 pm; Melodie has agreed to pick her up at the airport. To avoid the rush hour traffic, Melodie is thinking of asking Lisa to take a taxi to her house.

The following conversation occurs within Melodie's mind. Lisa has no knowledge of this.

Melodie (enters the Drama as Victim): "Oh, no, I have to pick Lisa up right at rush hour traffic."

Switching to Persecutor, Melodie says: "What kind of friend is Lisa that she would make her flight plans to arrive at 5:00 pm on a Friday! She has no consideration for me. She's supposed to be my friend, too."

Switch to Victim: "If I don't pick up Lisa at the airport, she won't like me." (Here Melodie is trying to prevent someone from withdrawing love by doing the right thing that will prevent this withdrawal. The Victim is at the mercy of the Other.) "Besides, I should be more caring. She has done so much for me."

Switch to Persecutor (of self): "What kind of friend am I that I can't even drive in traffic to pick up a friend who is so good to me?"

Switch to Rescuer (of Lisa): "Poor Lisa, she comes all this way and I make her take ground transportation."

Around and around Melodie went until, at last, she paused, took a deep breath and became aware that she was going around and around, over and over the same territory and getting nowhere. This awareness became the signal that she was Dancing the Drama.

Once aware, Melodie moved into Three Turns of the Kaleidoscope for Healing The Victim Within:

She started with the Six-Pointed Star Meditation.

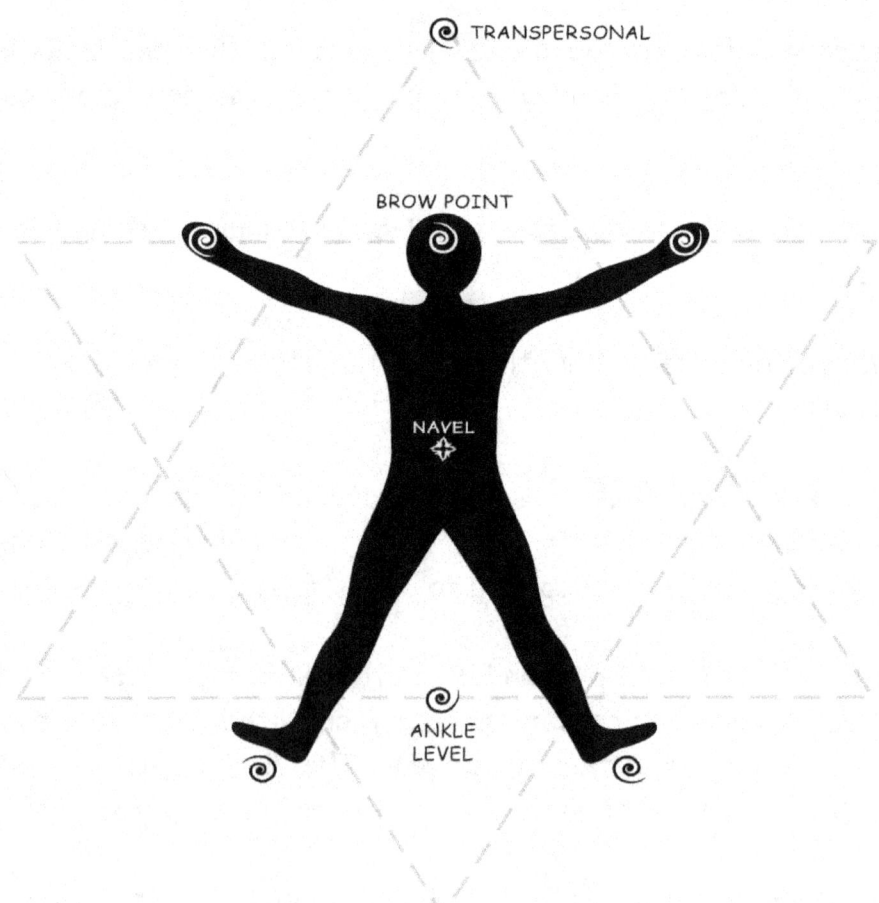

Then, she diagrammed the Drama Dance.

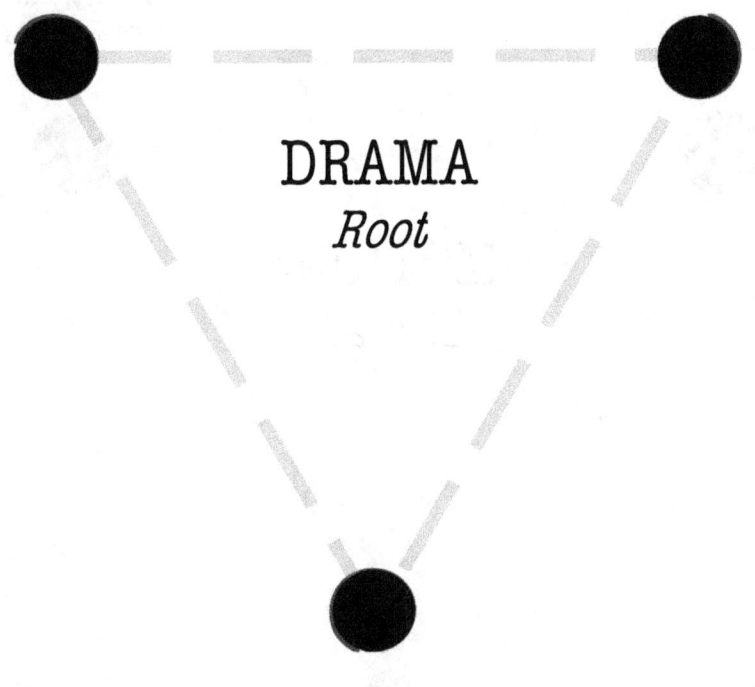

RESCUER

"Poor Lisa, she comes all this way and I make her take ground transportation."

PERSECUTOR

"What kind of friend am I that I can't even drive in traffic to pick up a friend who is so good to me?"

DRAMA
Root

VICTIM

"If I don't pick up Lisa at the airport, she won't like me."

Next she moved through the Need-Help-Action Triangle, asking herself the questions that revealed that she was scared and felt unsafe to tell Lisa to take a taxi. The transformational quality of Truth provided the help to perceive both the need and the action.

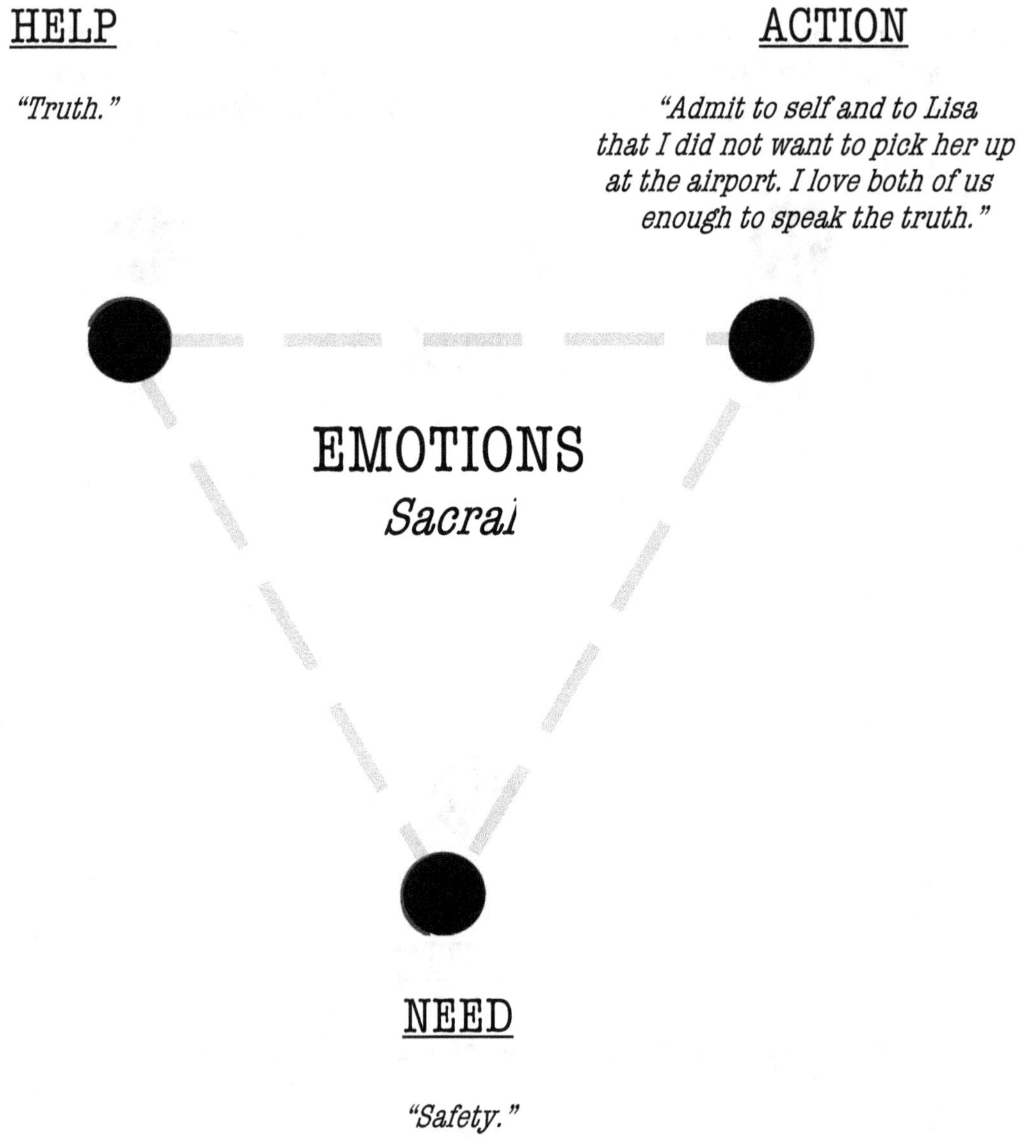

HELP

"Truth."

ACTION

"Admit to self and to Lisa that I did not want to pick her up at the airport. I love both of us enough to speak the truth."

EMOTIONS
Sacral

NEED

"Safety."

Next: Student-Teacher-Knowledge. Truth was her helper in this triangle also. Truth helped her to see that she still had a belief and a pattern of living in which her behaviors determined whether she was loved or unloved. In this Drama, she looked through the garbled lens and saw herself as conditionally loved. This put her in the awful position of having to behave in certain ways in order to meet the perceived conditions for remaining loved. Notice how this belief harkens back to the domestication process of rewards for good behaviors and punishment for bad behaviors.

KNOWLEDGE

*"Something inside of me
Still experiences love as conditional."*

THOUGHTS
Solar Plexus

STUDENT

"I am."

TEACHER

"Lisa."

Next: Death-Birth-Life Triangle   With the knowledge in hand, the next triangle was easy.   With this turn of the kaleidoscope, a major shift occurred. Through this kaleidoscope lens — crystal clear — she was able to perceive that seeking love that is conditional sets her up for receiving immature and undeveloped love; mature love is never conditional; the very definition of love forbids conditions*.

Prior to this shift, she had a cognitive awareness of loving herself and had many ways in which she did loving actions for herself. With this shift, loving herself – all of her – became as natural as breathing. Therefore, this realization transformed her.

LIFE

"I actively love me unconditionally."

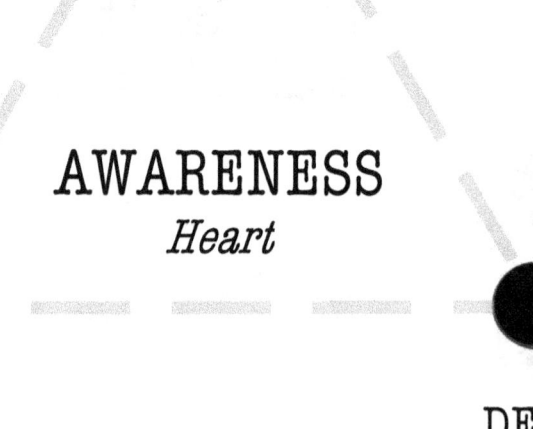

AWARENESS
Heart

BIRTH   DEATH

"Mature love is unconditional."   *"False belief that love is conditional."*

Loving herself is just as natural as breathing! Sometimes natural breathing is long and deep, sometimes shallow and quick, sometimes uneven, sometimes smooth.

*Setting and agreeing on certain conditions that help us relate, live and work well together is necessary and wise. For example, two people agree that they will each contribute fifty percent to the monthly food bill. This is the condition they both agree on to cooperatively share in buying food. They may express love for each other through this agreement. However, their love for each other is not dependent on this condition. If one person consistently neglects to pay their share, the other person may decide to do something else about purchasing food. However, the love continues. In fact, the expression of the love may be to create a new agreement that harms neither party. Love that is conditional says: "In order for me to love you, you must meet certain conditions." Alternatively: "In order for you to love me, I must meet certain conditions." Both forms of conditional love are immature and harmful to self, other and relationships.

NOTES:

Quick! What's Your First Thought?

Quick! What's your first thought when asked, "What is the need in this particular drama dance?" First thought?

Amazing, as it may seem, our first thoughts to the questions in the healing the Victim within process are usually the most accurate. By going with the first thought and quickly going on to the next questions in each of the healing triangles, one can go through the process in a short time and with internal changes that can be lived instead of analyzed. In addition, this "quick first thought" method usually bypasses or keeps at a minimum kindling, the hyper-arousal state of trauma that energizes the Drama Dance.

One of the best descriptions of how and why the first thought approach works is found in Malcolm Gladwell's book: *blink: The Power of Thinking Without Thinking*. Gladwell asserts: "…there can be as much value in the blink of eye as in months of rational analysis." He cites numerous research studies that elaborate, underscore, and support this premise. For example, "A person watching a two-second video clip of a teacher he or she has never met will reach conclusions about how good that teacher is that are very similar to those of a student who sat in the teacher's class for the entire semester."

Gladwell describes a part of our brain called "adaptive unconscious" that is "put to work …whenever we meet a new person or confront a complex situation or have to make a decision under stress." This "adaptive unconscious" is what produces that split-second information that is so often right information and right action. Often, this information feels like it has been pulled out of thin air.[62]

Physicist David Bohm describes the universe as a holomovement—a continuously moving hologram. One of the concepts of a hologram is that a minuscule "bite" of a hologram contains a picture of the whole in that bite.[63] This concept can be applied to the information gleaned with Gladwell's "blink of the eye" or "snap" judgment. The blink or snap contains the whole and one can confidently act on the information.

---

[62] Malcolm Gladwell pgs. 1-17
[63] Michael Talbot p.47

For the healing the Victim within process, the most significant and helpful information in Gladwell's findings revolves around this statement: "How good people's decisions are under the fast-moving, high-stress conditions of rapid cognition is a function of <u>training and rules and rehearsal</u>."[64]

This translates to mean that we can increase our accuracy in receiving blink-of-an-eye information and action through increasing our expertise in a particular arena. Gladwell describes how the more expertise a person, from food critics to basketball players, has in a certain area, the more effective they are. They are able to discern nuances in a tiny encounter that non-experts cannot come anywhere close to noticing.

For example, a nurse receives years of training, learns the basics of nursing, gets to know the rules, then practices the basics. With enough understanding and practice (rehearsals), the nurse develops into an expert. At the expert level, s/he assesses a situation, receives information in a blink of an eye and takes action. The nurse's accuracy at the expert level is greatly maximized compared to the neophyte nurse or layperson. Wise doctors know to pay attention when an expert nurse says: "I have a funny feeling about Joshua in room 10." Wise doctors act on that blink-of-an-eye information for the well being of Joshua.[65]

Let's take the example of a person who's Drama Dance is activated when trying to solve a conflict. The Drama internal dialogue might go like this: "If I tell John I resent it when he borrows my scissors without asking, he will probably yell at me. If he does that, I'll cry. If I cry, he'll stomp away, and then what will I do? I guess I won't say anything. He won't borrow them again. I know. I'll borrow his Ipod without asking. Then he'll get the message. What if he confronts me about borrowing his stuff? What will I say?"

This method is trying to predict ahead of time every conceivable verbal exchange. It is what is called plotting and planning. Based on mistrust of one's ability to think and act in the now, plotting and planning is a method for controlling for every conceivable possibility. Contrast this with training, rules, and rehearsals.

---

[64] Malcolm Gladwell pgs. 99-146

[65] Patricia Benner, pp. 13-34

Training, rules and rehearsals give the person in the above example a foundation for conflict resolution so that when she encounters a conflict, the skills for right word and right action arise easily and authentically. They arise in the now, not an artificial planned act. Training can be via attending a workshop, reading a book or watching a DVD on conflict resolution. The rules of conflict resolution can be learned. The skills and rules can be rehearsed in low stress environments. Friends with whom she has a high level of trust and safety can be enlisted to practice the skills. This all prepares her for spontaneous resolution of conflicts with information and action that have a greater potential of success.

Plotting and planning keeps one in the Victim mindset and is the Drama Dance. The process for healing the Victim within is training, with rules and rehearsals for living authentically in the now.

This could mean the more we practice the Three Turns of the Kaleidoscope, the more accurate will be our "Quick! First thought" responses.
Learning and practicing increases our expertise in encountering situations that previously catapulted us into the Drama Dance. This expertise provides blink-of-an-eye information that more accurately guides us to act for our greater good. We can perceive the Drama Dance potential and choose to move right to "What is my need here? What action? What help? What's the knowledge? What new has been created in me that I can choose to live right now?"

As we become more practiced and knowledgeable in this healing process, the accuracy of the "blink" information increases. Applying the healing the Victim within process to even minor Drama Dances provides more opportunities for rehearsals. Increased practice can move us toward greater ease in avoiding the Drama Dance and greater ease in choosing to peer through the crystal clear lens of the kaleidoscope.

NOTES:

Complete Step-By-Step Overview
Three Turns of a Kaleidoscope: Healing Victim Within

Prep 1: Invoking the healing energy of six-pointed star

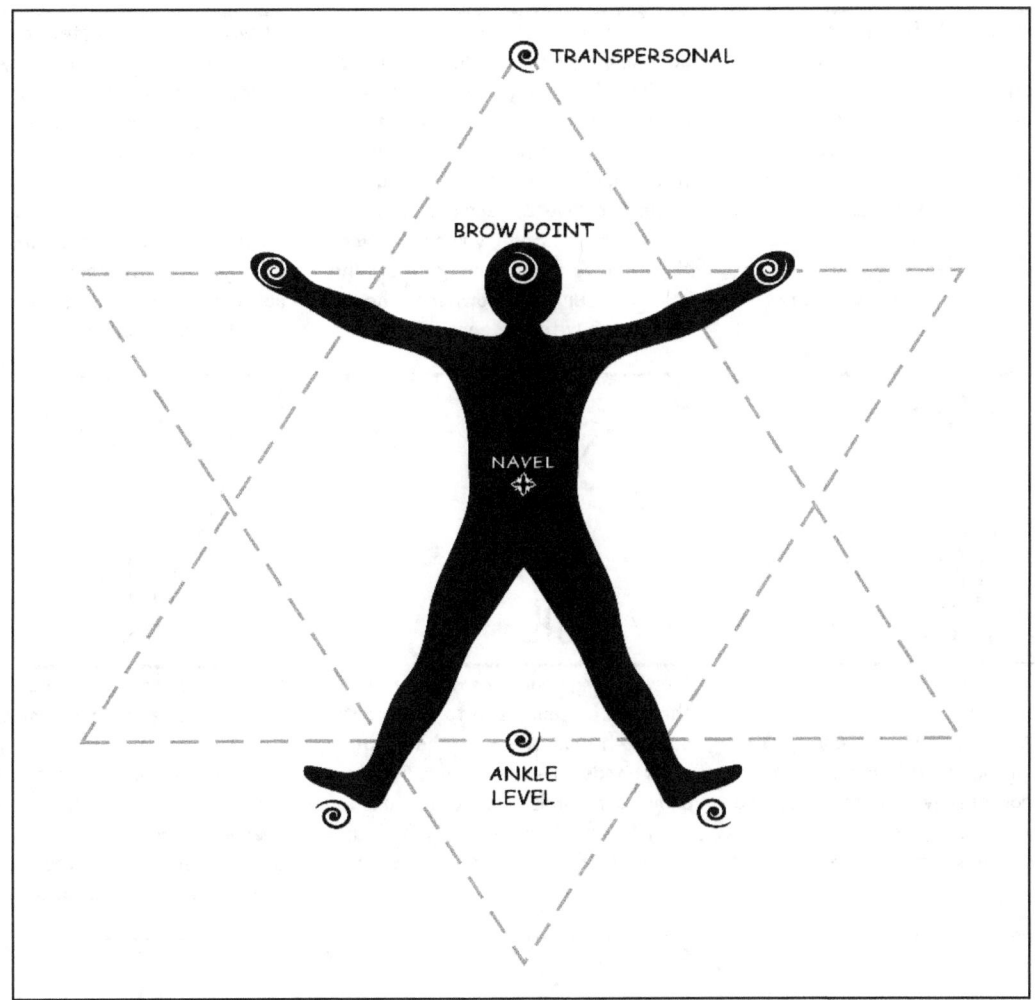

Locate the chakras or energy centers on the diagram and on yourself: the palms of the hands, the soles of the feet, the brow – front and back, the chakra at the level of the ankles, the transpersonal, and the navel. Notice the configuration of the six-pointed star is within the human energy system that extends about three feet beyond the physical body. Using a violet marker, complete or trace the star on the paper.

Next, trace the star in your human energy system by following the directions:

Six Pointed Star Meditation

1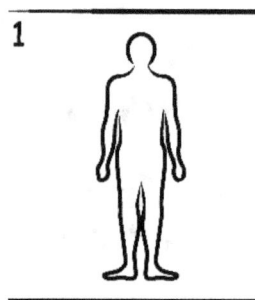

Prepare yourself for meditation by creating a space with as few distractions as possible. Sit or stand in a way that is physically comfortable for you. Let your attention move to your mid-chest. Quietly, observe yourself, breathing in and breathing out. No need to change your breathing. Just notice your breathing for a few minutes.

2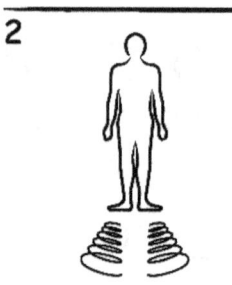

Gently, move your attention to the bottom of your feet. Become aware of the soles of your feet. Notice or imagine the energy centers at the bottom of your feet. Imagine that these moving vortexes of energy begin to activate, becoming stronger and stronger. Soon, you may notice the spinning flow reaching, from the soles of your feet, down into the ea resonating with the earth energies.

3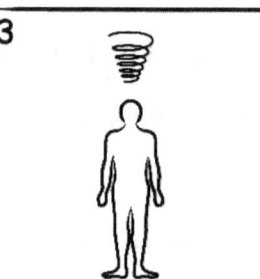

Slowly, move your attention to a spot about 18 inches above your head, letting your attention remain on this spot, known as the transpersonal energy center. Become aware of this energy center as a vortex of energy. Notice as it begins to activate, becoming stronger and stronger, flowing upward to the sun and resonating with the sun energies.

4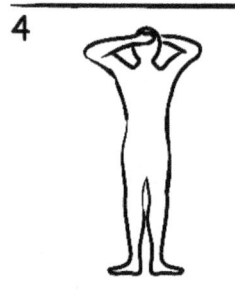

Place one hand on your brow, and the other hand on the back of your head. Allow life's healing energies to come through your hands and into your brow energy centers, front and back. Let yourself observe the brow energies for a minute.

5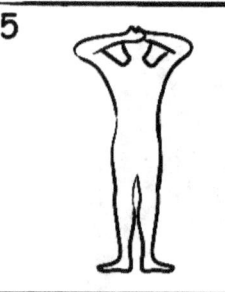

Slowly bring your rear hand from the back of your head to the front, putting it over the other hand so both hands cover the brow. Gently allow your hands to separate and move horizontally as far away from the midline of your body as possible.

6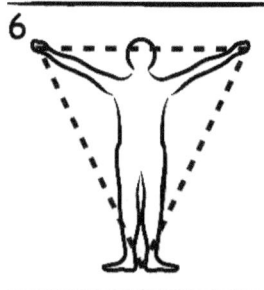

Your hands, following a horizontal energetic line, will be completely out to your sides and level with your brow. Then, pointing your hands down toward the ground, trace the energetic lines, toward the space between and beyond your feet. This forms the first energetic triangle.

7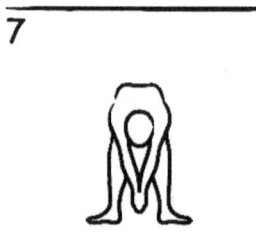

Place both hands into the space between your ankles, allowing the healing energies to come through your hands and into this space that is also an energy center. Gently allow your hands to separate and move horizontally.

8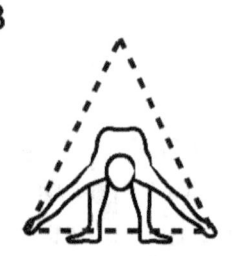

With your hands out as far away from your feet as possible, move your hands diagonally upward toward the ceiling/sun, meeting at a point over your head. You have traced the lines that form the second energetic triangle.

9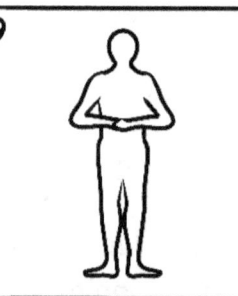

Move both hands to the navel, allowing the healing energies to come through your hands and into this powerful energy vortex. Rest in this awareness.

© 2008 Three Turns of a Kaleidoscope by Bonnie Johnson – Permission granted to duplicate for personal and educational purposes.

Prep 2: Remembering our Healthy Natural Mammal

1. Complete the drawing of Natural Mammal Triangle.

2. Identify one Natural Mammal experience in your own life. Briefly share with a trusted person. This could be with oneself verbally or symbolically

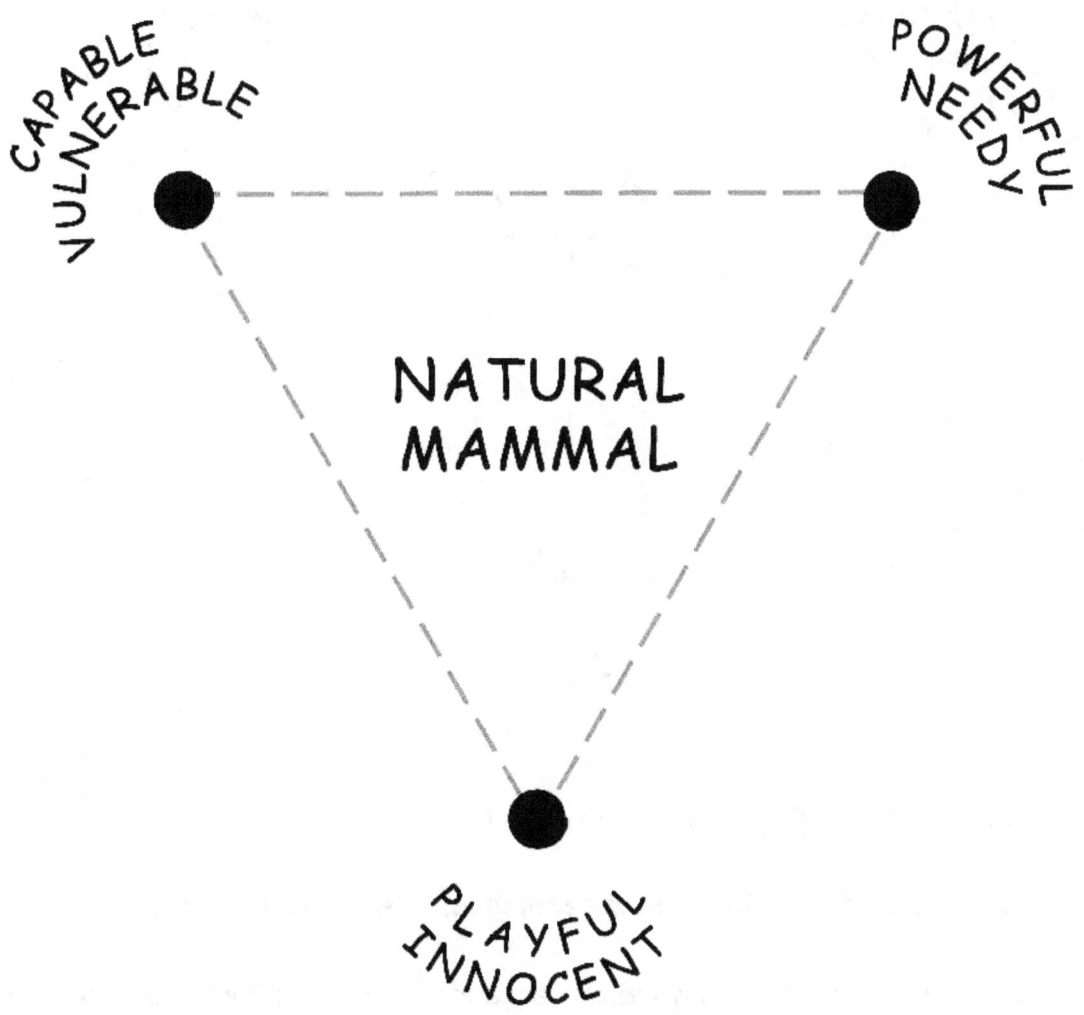

Prep 3: Choosing our Drama Dance experience

1. Repeat Six-Pointed Star Meditation.

2. Complete or Trace the drawing of the Victim-Rescuer-Persecutor Triangle.

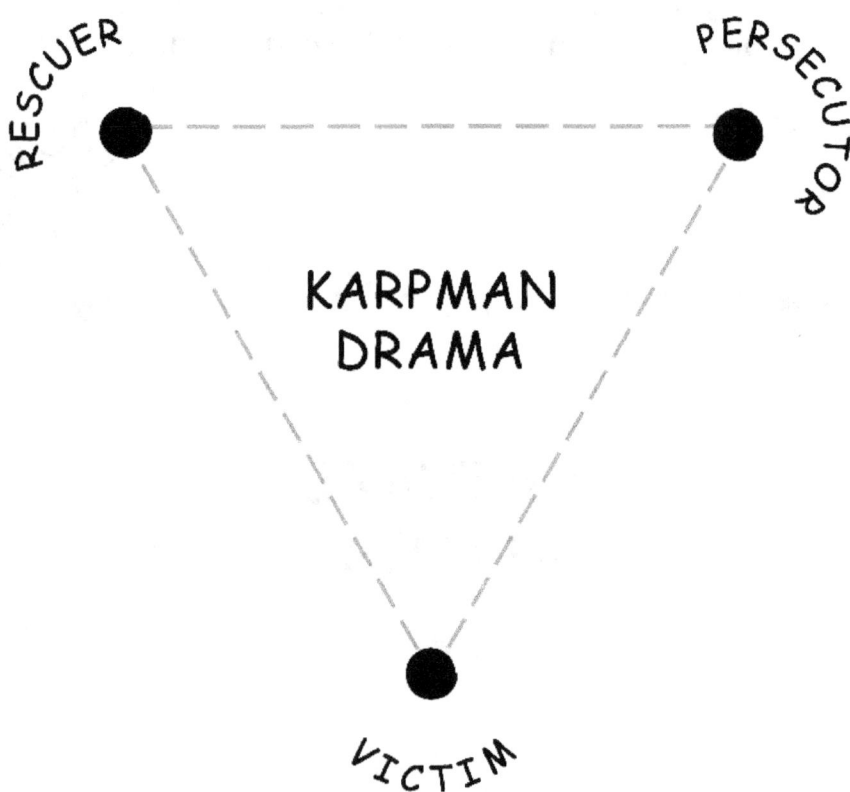

3. Choose a Drama Dance example in your life.

4. Experience an energetic healing technique. See pages 117-132.

5. Identify and write down a word or sentence that describes you in each of the roles. See "Tips On Identifying The Three Roles" on page 59.

6. Record this information the VRP drawing.

First Turn: Becoming safe

1. Complete the Need-Help-Action Triangle drawing.

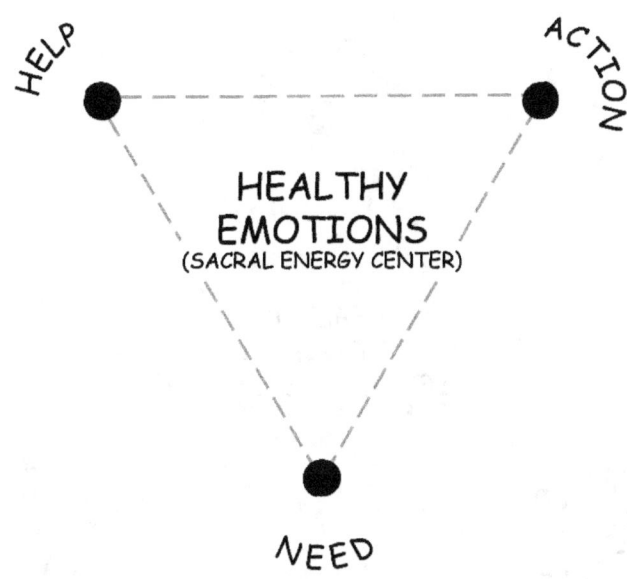

2. Repeat the Six-Pointed Star Meditation.
3. Use your Drama experience to:
   - **Identify the Need.** When we step onto the Drama Dance (DD) floor, what need are we trying to meet? The answer to the question has something to do with safety, survival, security, trust, and vitality.
   - **Identify the Help.** Examine what help is required to meet the identified need. Choose from transformational qualities: self-love, forgiveness or truth.
   - **Identify the Action.** Ask what action is needed to meet the identified need with help of the identified quality. Note: Answer with first thought.
4. Choose a word or sentence that encapsulates your answers. Record this information on the NHA drawing.
5. Experience an energetic healing technique as needed. (See pages 117-132.)

© 2008 Three Turns of a Kaleidoscope by Bonnie Johnson – Permission granted to duplicate for personal and educational purposes.

Second Turn: Shifting awareness to learning

1. Complete Student-Teacher-Knowledge Triangle drawing.

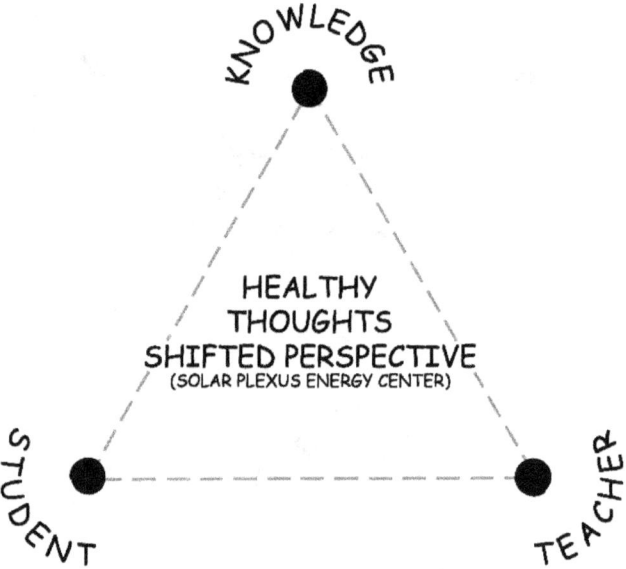

2. Repeat Six-Pointed Star Meditation.

3. In your Drama experience:
   - Identify the Student by asking, "Who is the Student?"
   - Identify the Teacher by asking, "Who is the Teacher?"
   - Discover the Knowledge by asking, "What am I learning from the teacher when I dance this drama?"

4. Choose a word or sentence that encapsulates your answers.

5. Record this information on the STK drawing

6. Experience an energetic healing technique as needed. (See pages 117-132.)

© 2008 Three Turns of a Kaleidoscope by Bonnie Johnson – Permission granted to duplicate for personal and educational purposes.

Third Turn: Transforming to living anew

1. Complete the Death-Birth-Life Triangle drawing.

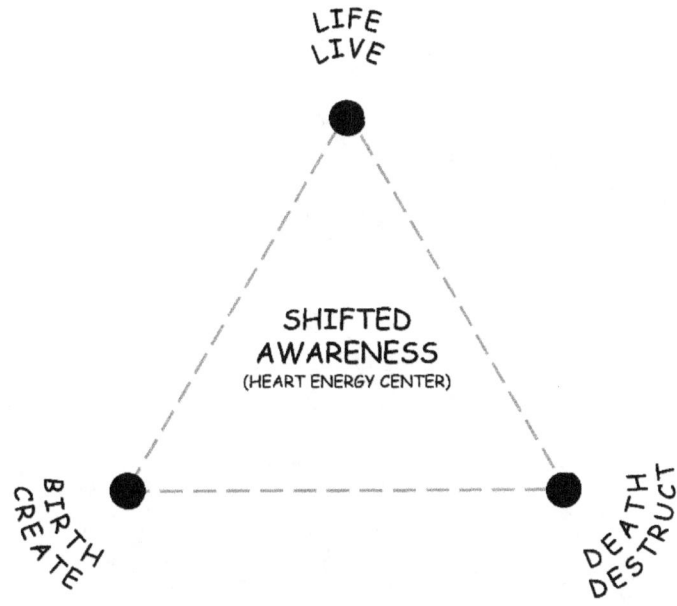

2. Repeat the Six-Pointed Star Meditation.
3. In your Drama experience:
   - Identify the Death by asking, "What in me is ready to destruct?"
   - Identify the Birth by asking, "What in me, is ready to be created?"
   - Reap the Living by asking, "What will that look like in my day to day life?"
4. Reinforce the Living: place one hand on your Heart Chakra and one on your Brow. Allow the Universal Healing Energies to infuse through your hands and into the two chakras. Allow Compassion, Wisdom and Higher Purpose to fill your heart and the new awareness.
5. Choose a word or sentence that encapsulates your answers.
6. Record this information on the DBL drawing

Now Celebrate!

NOTES:

BIBLIOGRAPHY

Spiritual Insights & Higher Consciousness:

Benner, Patricia. From Novice to Expert: excellence and power in clinical nursing practice (Menlo Park: Addison-Wesley, 1984)

Chopra, Deepak. Life After Death (New York: Harmony Books, 2006)

Gaffney, Mark H. *Gnostic Secrets Of The Naassenes* (Rochester, Vermont: Inner Traditions, 2005)

Gladwell, Malcolm. *blink: The Power Of Thinking Without Thinking* (New York: Little, Brown and Company, 2005)

Harvey, Andrew. *The Return Of The Mother* (New York: Penguin/Putnam, Inc, 1995)

Herbert, Nick. *Quantum Reality* (New York: Anchor Books, 1985)

Karon, Jan. *Light From Heaven* (New York: Viking Press, 2005)

Kenyon, Tom. *The Ghandarva Experience* (USA: S.E.E. Publishing Co. 1996)

Kincannon, Karla. *Creativity And Divine Surprise* (Nashville, Tennessee: Upper Room Books, 2005)

Leloup, Jean-Yves English translation and notes by Joseph Rowe. *The Gospel According To Mary Magdalene* (Rochester, Vermont: Inner Traditions, 2002)

MacEowen, Frank. *The Mist-Filled Path* (Novato, California: The New World Library, 2002)

Moore, Thomas. *Care of the Soul* (New York: HarperCollins *Publishers*, 1992)

Nepo, Mark. *The Exquisite Risk* (New York: Three Rivers Press/Random House, 2005)

Newberg MD, Andrew, D'Aquill MD, Eugene and Rause, Vince. *Why God Won't Go Away* (New York: Ballantine Books, 2001)

Palmer, Parker. *Hidden Wholeness* (San Francisco, California: Jossey-Bas, 2004)

Peat, F David. *Blackfoot Physics* (Grand Rapids, Michigan: Phanes Press, Inc, 2002)

Peat, F David. *Synchronicity* (New York: Bantam Books, 1987)

Pearce, Joseph Chilton. *Magical Child* (New York: Penguin Press, 1992)

Spiritual Insights & Higher Consciousness (con't):

Rice, David L. *Do Animals Have Feelings Too?* (Nevada City, California: Dawn Publications, 1999)

Rohr, Richard. *Adam's Return* (New York: The Crossroad Publishing Company, 2004)

Ruiz, Don Miguel. *The Four Agreements* (San Rafael, California: Amber-Allen Publishing, Inc., 1997)

Ruiz, Don Miguel. *The Mastery of Love* (San Rafael, California: Amber-Allen Publishing, Inc., 1999)

Schneider, Michael. *A Beginner's Guide To Constructing The Universe* (New York: HarperCollins Publishers, Inc, 1995)

Sheppard, Kay. *Food Addiction: The Body Knows* (Deerfield Beach, Florida: Health Communications, Inc, 1993)

Smith, Alexander McCall. *The Full Cupboard Of Life* (New York: First Anchor Books, 2005)

Starbird, Margaret. *Magdalene's Lost Legacy* (Rochester, Vermont: Bear & Company, 2003)

Starhawk. *Dreaming The Dark* (Boston: Beacon Press, 1982, 1988, 1997)

Talbot, Michael. *The Holographic Universe* (New York: HarperCollins Publishers, 1992)

Zafon, Carlos Ruiz translated by Lucia Graves. *Shadow Of The Wind* (New York: Penguin Books, 2004)

http://www.cduniverse.com/search/xx/music/pid/1008570/a/Rosa+Mystica.htm

Energetic Healing:

Brennan, Barbara. *Hands Of Light* (New York: Pleiades Books, 1987)

Bruyere, Rosalyn. *Wheels Of Light* (New York: Simon & Shuster, 1990)

Chia, Mantak. *Awaken Healing Energy Through The Tao* (New York: Aurora Press, 1983)

Eden, Donna with Feinstein, David. *Energy Medicine* (New York: Jeremy P. Tarcher/Putnam, 1999)

Gerber, Richard. *Vibrational Medicine* (Santa Fe, New Mexico: Bear & Company, 1988)

Grauds, Connie and Childers, Doug. *The Energy Prescription* (New York: Bantam Dell, 2005)

Hover-Kramer, Dorothea. *Healing Touch* (New York: Delmar Publishers, 2002)

Krieger, Dolores. *Therapeutic Touch* (New York: Simon & Schuster, 1979)

Energetic Healing (con't):

Leadbeater, C.W. *Chakras* (Wheaton, Illinois: The Theosophical Society in America, 1987)

Markides, Kyriacos C. *Fire In The Heart* (USA: Penguin Press, 1992) out-of-print

Takahashi, Takeo. *Atlas Of The Human Body* (New York: Harper Collins Publishers, 1989)

www.healingtouchinternational.org

www.sacred-geometry.com/sacredgeometry

www.therapeutictouch.org

www.rosalynlbruyere.org

www.innersource.net/energy_medicine

Transactional Analysis and Karpman Drama Triangle

Berne, Eric. *Games People Play* (New York: Ballantine Books, 1964, 1992)

Steiner, Claude. *Scripts People Live* (New York: Grove Press, 1974, 1990)

Stewart, Ian and Joines, Vann. *TA Today* (England and North Carolina: Lifespace Publishing, 1987, 2005)

www.ericberne.com

www.itaa-net.org/TAJNet/articles/karpman

www.coachingsupervisionacademy.com/our_approach/karpman_drama_triangle

www.karpmandramatriangle.com/pdf/dramatriangleupdate2007

www.KarpmanDramaTriangle.com

www.wikipedia.org/wiki/Karpman_drama_triangle

http://www.lynneforrest.com/html/the_faces_of_victim.html

Healing Trauma:

Ackerman, Diane. *Deep Play* (New York: Vintage Books, 1999)

Bryant, Roberta Jean. "The Magic of Profound Self-Acceptance" LOTUS, spring 1993 p. 38; excerpted from Stop *Improving Yourself And Start Living* (San Rafael, California: New World Library, 1991)

Grubin, David. *The Secret Life Of The Brain, Episode 4* (New York: PBS Home Video, 2001)

Hammerschlag, Carl. *The Theft Of The Spirit* (New York: Fireside Simon & Schuster, Inc, 1994)

Levine, Peter. *Healing Trauma* (Boulder, Colorado: Sounds True, Inc, 2005)

Levine, Peter *Waking The Tiger* (Berkeley, California: North Atlantic Books, 1997)

Miller, Alice – translated by Andrew Jenkins – *The Body Never Lies* (New York: WW Norton & Co, 2005)

Naparstek, Belleruth. *Invisible Heroes* (New York: Bantam Dell, 2004)

Remen, Rachel Naomi. *Kitchen Table Wisdom* (New York: Riverhead Books, 1996)

Scaer, Robert. *The Trauma Spectrum* (New York: W. W. Norton & Company, Inc., 2005)

Whitfield MD, Charles L. *Healing The Child Within* (Deerfield Beach, Florida: Health Communications, Inc., 1989)

Dictionaries

Merriam-Webster's Collegiate Dictionary, Tenth Edition (Springfield, Massachusetts: Merriam-Webster, Incorporated, 1999)

www.wikipedia.org

Acknowledgments

Writing about healing is completely different than being a healer or teaching about healing. For me, healing is easy and effortless. Sometimes even the actual writing slipped out of me and onto the page. Ah! But the revising that was a completely different animal. As I wrestled with the revisions, many people gave me critical support. Their insights, editing skills, and knowledge of clear writing helped immensely.

Special thanks to Lois Schmidt who read many of the original drafts and who did not shrink from giving plainspoken critiques, often in the form of "This doesn't make any sense." She willingly spent long periods of time analyzing and discussing a thought, sentence and pages until I understood just what was needed. Lois and E. H. "Buddy" Mason kept "my feet to the fire" in the seemingly endless manifestations of the Introduction. Buddy insistently and lovingly challenged me with "Give me a picture of what you are talking about. Write so I can see it in my mind." What deep gratitude I have for their not allowing me to settle for less than my best writing.

For their generous time and superb observations, I thank Harvey Baker, Elaine Benson, Grantham Couch, Pat Floyd, Karla Kincannon, Marty Rather and Vicki Slater. My journey of writing has been lightened by their presence.

Brian Parker, graphic artist extraordinaire, filled the illustrations with laughter, sharp wit and heart overflowing with love. What a pleasure were the hours we spent discussing and deciding on the illustrations.

Mary Catharine Nelson, my author representative from Westview publishing, thank you for literally holding my hand through the publishing process. Because of you, getting from writing to published has actually been fun.

Bounteous appreciation goes to Sheilah Winn for the use of her beautiful Florida beach house. As I wrote the first draft I experienced endless joy overlooking the glistening crystals of ocean and sun.

About the Author

A gifted and wise healer, Bonnie Johnson brings together a lifetime of experiences and transcends them into wisdom, all for the purpose of helping others to heal.

As nurse healer, teacher and writer, she draws on over forty-five years of professional experience in nursing, counseling and educating adults and children. In her holistic nursing practice, Bonnie provides and teaches hands-on energetic healing to individual clients, health care professionals and laypersons. In addition, she taught and supervised holistic nursing students in their field placements, serving as adjunct faculty at Tennessee State University's master level holistic nursing program.

She provides a healing ministry to members of her church community as well as teaches healing and leads healing services at churches and ecumenical retreat centers.

For over twenty years, she has studied spirituality, holistic nursing and healing through the international Healing Touch Certificate Program, Therapeutic Touch Professional Associates, American Holistic Nurses Associations and the Healing Light Center, She is a Registered Nurse (New England Deaconess School of Nursing), Certified Healing Touch Practitioner and Instructor, Certified Holistic Nurse, and Master's prepared Child Development Specialist (George Peabody College); and has studied religion at Scarritt College graduating with a BA in Behavioral Sciences.

Her writings have appeared in *Tennessee Nurse* and *School Age Notes*, the international newsletter for school-age care professionals where she was the editorial manager for eleven years. Her multimedia presentation: *Telling Our Story: Holistic Nursing and Healing* has been a keynote feature at the annual conferences of the Tennessee Nurses Association, Healing Touch International, and the American Holistic Nurses Association. Her children's story (*What would you do if Sammy hit you?*) was broadcast on Arkansas radio.

In her healing work, Bonnie is guided and supported by the spiritual presence and counsel of Mary Magdalena whom she first communicated with as a three year old growing up in a small Massachusetts city. Through this guidance, Bonnie has developed many energetic healing techniques, including the Six-Pointed Star Meditation, Three Gates and Three Cauldrons, the Amygdala Connection: calming the runaway heart, and the Chakra Correspondence.

Bonnie's philosophy of healing, which she lives and teaches, is that as we heal we are helping to heal others and the earth. She extends her healing efforts toward the earth by planting and protecting trees. An avid gardener of native plants and trees, Bonnie has created a haven for birds and wildlife at her Nashville, Tennessee home.

She is currently writing a novel of historical fiction based on the spirited lives of her Scottish grandparents.

www.ingramcontent.com/pod-product-compliance
Lightning Source LLC
Chambersburg PA
CBHW051210290426
44109CB00021B/2410